BLOKES INC.
PLAY A BIGGER GAME

A blueprint for a healthier and happier life

TORY TREWHITT

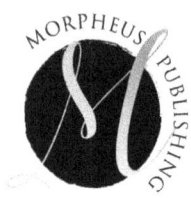

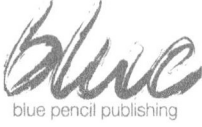

Copyright © 2025
First Published in Australia in 2025
By Morpheus Publishing
Geelong Victoria 3216
www.morpheuspublishing.com.au

All rights reserved. No part of this publication may be reproduced, stored in a retrieval system, or transmitted in any form or by any means, electronic, mechanical, photocopying, recording or otherwise, without the prior written permission of the publisher or author.

Paperback ISBN:	**9781764006316**
Author:	**Tory Trewhitt**
Senior Editor:	**Justine Martin**
Editor:	**Julie Athanasiou**
Cover Graphics:	**Lynette Ingles**

A catalogue record for this book is available from the National Library of Australia.

DISCLAIMER
The information contained in this book is for general informational purposes only. The author and publisher are not offering any medical, legal or professional advice. While every effort has been made to ensure the accuracy and completeness of the information provided, the author and publisher assume no responsibility for errors or omissions or any outcomes or consequences resulting from using this book's content.

COPYRIGHT
All original material in this book is the sole property of the author and Morpheus Publishing.

DISTRIBUTION
This book is distributed by Morpheus Publishing and is available through authorised distributors, booksellers, Morpheus Publishing website and Tory Trewhitt website.

COPYRIGHT PERMISSIONS
For copyright permissions or any other inquiries, please contact:
PUBLISHER: Morpheus Publishing
www.morpheuspublishing.com.au || hello@justinemartin.com.au || +61403 564 942

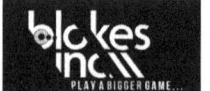

AUTHOR: Tory Trewhitt
https://torytrewhitt.com.au/ || info@trewhealth.com.au
https://www.morpheuspublishing.com.au/authors/tory-trewhitt

DEDICATION

To the incredible team at Blokes Inc.,

Thank you for your unwavering support, inspiration, and partnership. Your dedication to excellence, creativity, and pushing boundaries has been a constant source of motivation. The collaboration we've shared has been nothing short of amazing, and I am deeply grateful for every challenge, idea, and conversation that has shaped this journey.

To my parents, Graeme and Joan, your unwavering love, guidance, and support have been the foundation of who I am today. You've always been there for me, no matter where life took me, regardless of my mood (especially during my more challenging moments). Your belief in me has never wavered, and I am forever grateful for everything you've done. Who would have thought I'd become an author?

To my sisters, Shelli and Lara, thank you for shaping me as your baby brother, for being a constant source of love and strength, and for helping me grow in ways only siblings can.

To Gerard McMahon, a great sounding board and brother-in-law, your attention to detail and your feedback—especially when I was exhausted from reading my work—has been invaluable. You've been a key part of this journey, and I can't thank you enough.

To Julie Athanasiou, your editing skills have brought this project to life, and your expertise and patience mean the world.

To Juzzy Martin and her amazing publishing team, thank you for enduring my countless changes. Your professionalism and dedication were instrumental in getting this project over the finish line, but the journey has just started!

To Andrew Jobling, my friend, mentor, and accountability coach for the past 20 years. You've helped me push beyond my limits, and I could not have completed this without your wisdom and encouragement.

To my incredible clients over the past 20 years—your challenges, inspiration, and motivation have driven me to be better, to do better, and to never stop learning. Thank you for pushing me toward the person I am today.

To my wife, Fiona, and my three beautiful kids, Indie, Tommy, and Billy—your love, support, and daily inspiration fuel everything I do. You are the reason I get up at 5 am, drink caffeine, and continue to dream big. Behind every good person is a great team, and you all mean the world to me.

And last but not least, to all the POBS (Peninsula Old Boys) and honorary POBS—what an incredible group of people you are. I am beyond thankful for your friendship, love, and support. During many tough years I knew I had the backing of so many good people even if I don't show it. My journey as a boy, teenager, adult, husband and father would not have been possible without each and every one of you. Thank you.

With all my love and gratitude,

TT

Life is a journey—you can't control the start, but you can control the finish.

—**Tory Trewhitt**

FOREWORD
by Michael Klim

I vividly remember having a colourful discussion with my personal trainer and good friend Tory Trewhitt about one of our most passionate subjects—men's health and why the average man is in total denial about facing up to their health issues.

Tory quoted Henry David Thoreau: 'Why do the "mass of men lead such quiet lives of desperation"? Come on, Kimmy, how many men do you know that are genuinely happy?'

That got me thinking, and although I considered myself to be a happy, cheerful man, I had to admit that in 2020, when I was diagnosed with chronic inflammatory demyelinating polyneuropathy. This autoimmune disorder significantly affected my body, and my life changed dramatically. Suddenly, I was faced with a new reality—one where I was no longer invincible. I, too, became depressed and noticed how many other men also looked sad and depressed.

As an athlete, I had spent years chasing the black line at the bottom of the pool, focusing on one goal: finishing first. My life revolved around swimming, and for many years, that single-minded dedication led me to the ultimate success. I had competed in three Olympic Games and achieved six Olympic Games medals, the most prominent being the Sydney 4x100 m gold medal over the USA, who threatened to 'smash us like guitars.' I also had 11 Commonwealth Games medals, 26 World Championship medals, and 20 aquatic world records.

However, in my darkest days of rehabilitation, I realised that my approach to health had to evolve. Being physically strong was no longer enough. I needed to become multi-dimensional, to holistically nurture my body, mind and spirit. That's where Blokes Inc. came into my life, having worked with Tory in the corporate health sector as a keynote speaker for his business. Together, we preached about the importance of becoming multi-dimensional, looking after your mental health, and establishing mindfulness practices (surfing, drawing, playing the guitar, meditation, and so forth). I realised it was now time for me to practice what I preached.

The knowledge that Tory and I shared with others provided me with the framework that helped me navigate this challenging journey. This self-exploration exposed my vulnerability, and I realised the importance of communication, particularly with the loved ones that matter. Tory's lessons in *Blokes Inc. Play a Bigger* Game highlight that looking after one's health daily is non-negotiable.

After my diagnosis, I initially neglected my health. I became angry, disillusioned, and fell into the 'why me' mindset. I threw away the tools that made me a world champion and successful businessman. Then, through the support of my friends and, more importantly, my partner Michelle and the kids, I reverted to my old habits around health and fitness. I realised that the strategies I had relied on during my 20-year professional athlete career could help me turn my situation around.

These strategies included:
- returning to healthy habits
- using exercise to help my body perform at its best
- building a solid nutritional platform
- prioritising rest and recovery.

I am constantly challenged to this day, but as Tory says, the key ingredient is consistency, so I can't encourage you enough to act, take control, and start the journey.

Tory's passion shines through every chapter, and it's clear that the challenges he's faced transitioning from health to hospitality have shaped the incredible insights he shares. *Blokes Inc. Play a Bigger Game* doesn't just offer lessons; it educates, motivates, and inspires with practical tools and tips that have been invaluable in my recovery. I still watch the *30 Days to Wellness* videos Tory created, and they remain a cornerstone of my daily routine. I hope you enjoy my input!

I wholeheartedly recommend *Blokes Inc. Play a Bigger Game* as it is a book that will empower you to invest in your health and remind you that taking care of yourself is one of the most important commitments you can make.

Over the years, I've worked alongside Tory with his corporate health business. It was a privilege, and we still enjoy working together today. We have both learnt valuable lessons from each other as friends, fathers, partners, business owners and health enthusiasts. Still, his passion and enthusiasm to help others is infectious and sets him apart. I was fortunate enough to read the first draft of *Bloke Inc. Play a Bigger Game* and agree with Tory that getting men physically and mentally fit with the right attitude is the first step to living a happier and healthier life.

What stands out to me about *Blokes Inc. Play a Bigger Game* is that, finally, there is a solution that most men can relate to. They can do it themselves, with their mates, or even better, with a group of blokes who can help keep them accountable. Together, they can change their mindset, face their pain points, learn, educate, and motivate themselves to live a happier and healthier life.

I love the book; the real stories, the real-life solutions, and the importance of running your body like a business make perfect sense. The chapter on bio-individuality is one of my favourites, as it explains that everyone is different. They have different goals, expectations, and ambitions and their programs need to reflect this. Jake's story in Chapter

12 was my favourite because I could deeply relate. The fear of failure and the internal mental dialogue that comes with it resonated with me.

Indeed, *Blokes Inc. Play a Bigger Game* is not only educational, but it also has plenty of inspirational stories and practical solutions. If nothing else, it reminds you that taking care of yourself is one of the most important commitments you can make.

Well done, TT. I am super proud of you, and it's been a pleasure to have a little input into your journey as an author. Who would have thought that our friendship would evolve from the gym floor to climbing mountains in Tassie, educating and motivating corporates around the importance of health, creating wellness weekends and retreats, and now both becoming published authors?

MICHAEL KLIM
#MK

TABLE OF CONTENTS

DEDICATION III

FOREWORD VII
  by Michael Klim

CHAPTER 1 1
  About Blokes Inc.

CHAPTER 2 23
  Motivation, mindset and habits

CHAPTER 3 45
  Nutrition and improving your energy

CHAPTER 4 73
- Mastering nutrition: key principles for a balanced diet

CHAPTER 5 111
- The art of exercise

CHAPTER 6 137
- Know your numbers

CHAPTER 7 155
- Sleep is not a tradable commodity

CHAPTER 8 177
- That dirty word 'stress'

CHAPTER 9 197
- Social connectivity

CHAPTER 10 221
- Sex: The role of sex in health and relationships

CHAPTER 11 237
- Bio-individuality: one size does not fit all

CHAPTER 12 257
- Your legacy

REFERENCES 269

CHAPTER 1

Life is a game. You make the rules.

—**Tory Trewhitt**

Reflecting on where you are versus where you want to be

As you begin your journey to take control of your health, I want you to take a moment and reflect on where you stand right now—both physically and mentally. Now, imagine where you'd like to be in the near future. Is there a significant difference?

In this book, I will share my struggles, the dark moments that tested me and how I built a path back using a wellness platform and habit stacking. These tools helped me reclaim both my body and mind. But first, let me take you back to one of the most challenging days of my life.

A challenging day begins

It was Friday 6 November 2020, and honestly, it felt like Groundhog Day as I made my way to my restaurant. I didn't have time to reflect on Byron Bay's beauty; I was consumed with what had to be done for the day. I knew I would be busy, as I had reduced the staff roster to save money, meaning I only had one cook rostered on until 5 pm.

In the back of my mind, I thought, *it's a Friday; why am I putting myself under all this pressure?* Part of me knew there would be enough trade to cover the restaurant's costs, but in hospitality, you never know, so I took the conservative approach, which meant I would be doing everything: prepping, cutting fish, making salads, serving customers, and cleaning, all while trying to keep the customers happy and turn a profit before closing the doors later that night.

Before I started my day's work, my morning ritual was to stop for a shot of caffeine to elevate my enthusiasm. As I got closer to town, the main street slowly woke up. Tourists and locals alike ambled down the footpaths, ready to make the most of this little slice of paradise I now call home.

Beyond that peaceful collective, I saw fellow business owners opening for the day. Their purpose resonated with me: would it be a profitable day? With my double shot latte in hand, I arrived to start the morning prep, knowing that I had three hours until the first customer would order around 11 am. Before this, I had to filter the oil, make fresh salads, fillet and portion the snapper, barramundi and salmon, clean the grill, set up the shop, open the tills and pack the stock away for what would hopefully be the start of a busy weekend.

With a small restaurant in a tourist town, you must account for many daily variables, including the weather, staffing, tourism and, at this time, the COVID-19 pandemic. My daily ordering needed to be as accurate as possible to be cost-effective.

The downside of running the shop so lean was that if the previous day's trade was good, our fresh fish supplies could be low the next day. Also, today was a Friday, which meant a later delivery time as the businesses that usually get stock before us would have increased their ordering volume to accommodate the weekend's trade.

At 11 am, I opened for trading, the same time my first staff member, Veronica, the cook, would arrive. I had worked with Veronica for around eight months. She was a hard-working Argentinian, good under pressure when trade got busy and we worked well together.

Usually, once the restaurant was set up for service, I would continue doing the prep, take orders when a customer arrived, or answer the phone. At the same time, Veronica looked after all the cooking requirements. Once she checked the docket for take-away or dine-in, I would deliver, clean, serve and repeat. If trade was quiet, I would keep prepping.

On this particular Friday, we had a solid lunch trade, so after the lunch service, I still needed to cut the fish and set up the display fridges. Part of the shop's aesthetics was the salad and fresh fish display. Daily, we would display the six salads freshly made in the morning. Then, once the fish delivery arrived, I would fillet enough for the lunch trade and then hang a few salmon, snapper and barramundi bodies for the visual effect.

An unexpected injury

On this day, I was becoming frustrated that the fish hadn't arrived, and it was already close to 2 pm, well after the lunch rush. The later the delivery, the longer I would have to stay in the store as I was the only staff member who could competently portion fish bodies.

At last, I heard the fish delivery guy arrive and there was always some banter between us. I would express my frustration, 'that it was hard to run a fish shop with no fish,' and his response was always, 'Order more fish the day before, you tight arse.'

Nevertheless, the fish had arrived now, so I could start the filleting and preparing the display cabinet. On this day, I noticed as I lifted the salmon body onto the filleting bench that it was a big one, close to 8 kg, by my estimation.

I remember grasping the knife with my right hand as usual and committing a quick, firm blow to the salmon. At that moment, I wasn't fully aware of my action, but the knife must have been off-centre as it hit the salmon's body with unexpected force.

Instead of piercing the salmon tail, the knife slid down the side of the salmon's body and stopped when the knife hit the filleting bench. Due to the velocity of my action, my fingers followed the force of the knife and slid straight down the face of the blade.

In less than one second, I saw my three fingers peel off. There was blood but no pain as I had cut through everything. All the ligaments and tendons of my middle, ring and little finger was severed entirely. I had even cut through the bone of my little finger.

My first response was to grab a handful of ice out of the fish bin and wrap a tea towel around my bloodied hand. I knew it wasn't good; I didn't know if all three fingers were entirely on or off.

Panicked, I reached Veronica and said, 'I have just cut three fingers off!'

At times, my humour and the language barrier confused her, and this was another example as she smiled and laughed.

I said, 'No, I'm serious! I need to go to hospital.'

My expression must have been loud enough for a customer to hear and they could sense Veronica didn't understand my urgency.

I repeated to her, 'I have just cut three fingers off; I need to go to the hospital!'

I was ushered out to the back of the shop to the courtyard.

The universe must have been looking after me as, within two minutes, my wife, Fi, unexpectedly arrived at the restaurant.

She asked what I had done, and I replied, 'Cut three fingers off.' Her first response was explicative, as this was just another example of the business continually challenging us.

The shock initially kept me coherent, but I fell to my knees as I walked towards Fi's car. Things were starting to get serious as we proceeded to the hospital. Fi called ahead and warned emergency that we were on our way, explaining what had happened as numerous thoughts raced through my mind.

Would I only have a thumb and a pointer finger? Could they reattach the three fingers? How will I keep fit and lift weights if I only have a pointer and a thumb?

As we pulled into the emergency bay, a team of eight doctors and nurses were ready to act.

It all happened quickly from the car to a wheelchair to the emergency room. The fierce fluorescent lighting had a sobering impact as I lay in the Emergency Department. As the medical staff shuttled about, I started to think about what effect this injury would have on me, my family, my business—everything.

Surgery and the reality of recovery

Before long, the local doctor was on the phone with Tweed Heads Hospital up the highway, explaining the extent of my injury. The plastic surgeon from Tweed Heads laid out the next steps.

First, they would carefully remove the tea towel, clean the area as much as possible and assess the damage. Once the wound was visible, the plan was to take photos and send them to the surgeon. If it looked serious, I'd be rushed up the coast by ambulance for surgery.

I couldn't look as the nurses peeled away the tea towels. The image of my fingers sliding down the filleting knife was still too fresh. The room was packed—everyone except me seemed eager to see the damage. Conversations flew, medications were administered, photos were snapped and X-rays were taken.

Before I knew it, I was on my way to John Flynn Private Hospital on the Gold Coast for surgery.

When I arrived at John Flynn, my pain scale was now 11/10 as I paced around the waiting room, attempting to take my mind off it. Then, a nurse informed me that the surgeon was currently in the operating theatre, but I would be next.

The pain was becoming unbearable. After what felt like an eternity in the waiting room, a nurse noticed how much I was struggling and promised to contact the anaesthetist, who was in the operating theatre. The medical staff decided they would take me down immediately to insert a nerve block and prep me for surgery. A mix of nervousness, anxiety and relief flooded my mind as a nurse wheeled me deeper into the operating department.

In the pre-op area, the anaesthetist greeted me, calmly explaining the process before prepping the nerve block. He mentioned the surgeon would be along shortly to discuss the operation. Meanwhile, a nurse started cleaning and sterilising the area. Soon after, I felt the sting of the local anaesthetic as it was injected into my veins, followed by the nerve block. The initial sharp sensation was uncomfortable but brief.

As the anaesthetic spread through my system, I felt a stinging warmth, followed by a welcome numbness—finally, the pain started to fade.

I could feel my body relax, lying still on the theatre bench. Moments later, the surgeon rushed in, dressed in scrubs, gloves and a headlamp. The conversation was brief and straight to the point:

> *We have had a good look at the photos, X-rays and reports, and at this stage, we don't exactly know the extent of your injuries until we remove all the compression bandages. The good news is that you will be operated on shortly and the most extensive surgical operation I have done on someone's hand was a little over three hours. So, within that time, I will contact your wife and speak to you in recovery before discharge later today.*

Hearing the surgeon say the operation would only take three hours and that I'd be released the same day instantly shifted my mindset. There was a mix of relief and determination to tackle the recovery head on. I knew that my body would take a hit, but I also knew that my mindset would dictate how quickly I bounced back. Instead of dwelling on the discomfort or potential setbacks, I focused on what I could control. Staying positive, following the rehab process, and leaning into the same resilience I preach to others.

I remember waking up with a severe case of post-anaesthesia grogginess, accompanied by a bit of confusion, dizziness and a sense of nausea. With my blurred vision, I could see an arm pillow elevating my hand. I had a drip line inserted into my shoulder, which I later found out was morphine for self-administered pain relief.

Within a few minutes of waking, the nurse arrived for post-operative care, asked how I felt on the pain scale, took my blood pressure, observed other vital signs, and said the surgeon would be in within half an hour.

Enter the surgeon:

> *Tory, the surgery went well, but we didn't expect the extent of the damage that the accident caused. The operation took over six-and-a-half hours as we had to re-attach your ligaments and tendons and try to find another blood supply for your little finger. At this stage, we don't know if your little finger will survive as the blood flow has been severely compromised, but I advise you to abstain from coffee, alcohol and dark chocolate for at least four weeks. Should you observe any discolouration, please contact my rooms immediately. Otherwise, I will review your fingers in five days.*

Before I could ask any questions, he had left the room and I was left to digest the post-operative report myself.

Over the next 48 hours, I had to reach specific physiological markers. Two days later, I was finally discharged. The total cost of the operation was $41,000.

I learned that life could change quickly and that every action has consequences. At that time, I was temporarily physically disabled but mentally sharp and determined. My focus was on understanding the lessons from this experience and finding a way to transform a negative, traumatic event into a positive, career-defining opportunity.

Embracing rehabilitation and moving forward

Mastering my mental health was my initial focus before focusing on my future. Initially, I reflected on the 'why me' attitude. This business was the gift that kept on giving. The negative encounters just seemed to be stacking up one after the other.

I knew self-pity wasn't the answer, and if I was going to move forward, I needed clarity, focus and determination.

I started focusing on the little things every day that would aid my recovery. Consistency and structure would be the key ingredients, so I established a plan with my exercise physiologist background, surgeon and hand therapist.

Fortunately, Workcover allowed me an initial three-month treatment plan, so I didn't have to worry about my wage or rush back to work on light duties; I could dedicate my time to recovering. Unfortunately, there was still some uncertainty about my little finger and whether it would survive since it had limited blood supply for so long before surgery. Nevertheless, I intended to have five fingers rather than four, so I embraced the rehabilitation process.

The first few weeks of rehabilitation were a daze as I was in bed with my hand elevated in an arm elevation pillow to help reduce post-surgical swelling, along with a morphine intravenous line in my shoulder.

Five days after undergoing hand surgery, I returned for a post-operative check-up. The procedure involved internal and external stitches, carefully placed to address the injury. Upon inspection, the hand remained swollen, with the fingers puffy and immobilised, as if locked in a flexed position. Movement was severely limited, and any attempt to straighten the fingers was met with resistance.

Despite these challenges, the medical team reassured me that the swelling and rigidity were expected at this stage of recovery. The stitches, both beneath the skin and along the surface, held the surgical site securely as the healing continued.

Rehabilitation brought with it a host of psychological challenges that tested my resilience as much as the physical ones. The isolation was palpable; with little external support beyond sporadic phone calls from my case manager, I often felt alone in navigating this demanding journey.

Each day in rehab I pushed my body to its limits, forcing me to confront pain, discomfort, and the frustration of slow progress. Mentally, the battle was equally intense, fighting off doubts, staying motivated and managing the emotional weight of limited mobility. Yet, through it all, I remained steadfast, focusing on the long-term goal of regaining full use of my hand, removing myself from the hospitality industry and back into health and wellness, where I had worked for two decades prior to opening the restaurant.

That vision of recovery became my anchor, reminding me that each challenge I overcame was a step closer to the life I wanted to reclaim.

To this day, I am grateful that I can clench my fist, even if not perfectly. My little finger survived, and to the untrained eye, you would never know that I cut three fingers off in the blink of an eyelid. But life is not about perfection; it is about operating at your optimal level, and only you know what this looks like. So, many key learnings were the value of staying positive, plus recognising the importance of creating structure and consistency.

Never truly alone

This experience gave me a deeper understanding of how challenging life can be. But even in those suffocating, dark moments, we're never truly alone. The key to surviving these dark moments is finding the courage to take responsibility and seek help when needed. That's where *Blokes Inc. Play a Bigger Game* comes in—a reflection of my journey and the thousands of men I have helped.

For over two decades, I have dedicated my career to the health and fitness industry as an exercise physiologist, educator, motivator, strength and conditioning coach, and personal trainer. During this time, I have had the privilege of helping countless men overcome challenges such as addiction, chronic disease, lack of direction, career burnout, anxiety and depression.

Despite the diversity of their struggles, I have found that the formula for success remains consistent: fostering positivity, creating structured plans, maintaining consistency and ensuring accountability. This approach has empowered my clients to reclaim their health, find purpose and build sustainable, fulfilling lives.

Throughout my career, I have seen many blokes fall into the trap of becoming one-dimensional, pouring all their energy into their careers and financial pursuits under the belief that providing for their families is their sole priority. While their intentions are noble, this narrow focus often comes at a high cost, including strained relationships, declining health and, ultimately, lives that begin to unravel. Witnessing this has fuelled my passion for guiding men toward a more balanced, multidimensional approach to life. I passionately believe that health is the foundation upon which everything else is built. When men prioritise their physical and mental wellbeing, they can show up more fully in all areas of life at work, at home and in communities.

Life is a series of events, experiences, challenges and circumstances. We all face setbacks, but our reactions define what happens next.

Setting the foundation: nutrition, exercise and sleep

In *Blokes Inc. Play a Bigger Game*, chapter by chapter, I will focus on the critical ingredients for living a happier and healthier life. I believe the fundamentals for this are nutrition, exercise and sleep. But I will also cover the other aspects of life that will make you a multidimensional person. These bonus but vital elements are mindset, social connection, stress levels, bio-individuality, sex and your legacy.

Discovering what it truly means to thrive, *Blokes Inc. Play a Bigger Game* will guide you on a journey to better health and wellbeing in achievable and personal ways. You will find practical advice and straightforward strategies to empower you to make sustainable changes that work within your lifestyle. Whether you are looking to boost your energy, improve relationships or get a better handle on stress, each chapter provides insights that speak to your everyday needs. You will gain a deeper understanding of prioritising health and happiness—not by aiming for perfection, but by building habits that align with who you are and what you value.

Building change with the core trio: what, how and when

Each chapter includes the 'core trio' to making change happen—what, how and when. You need to include these elements in your plan to make real change. Using this core trio, you will start with minor improvements that will redefine what it means to be your best self. This might involve building healthier habits, creating a balanced lifestyle with daily rituals and mindfulness, spending more time with loved ones, lowering health risks like weight, blood pressure and cholesterol, or boosting your self-esteem.

For some, the change may be more significant. You might be considering a major life shift—moving to the coast or countryside, relocating overseas, switching careers or even starting your own business.

Whatever path you choose it must be driven by your intrinsic motivation to act now and make the change. *Blokes Inc. Play a Bigger Game* is here to help you take that first step. But remember, short-term actions bring short-term results. The number one ingredient in creating lasting change is consistency. Stay committed, and you'll see the transformation.

Why I am here to guide you

Why am I qualified to write about this? I have tried it, started it, sold it, failed at it, or am still looking for it. As a 'serialpreneur' (much to my wife's frustration), Blokes Inc. has been 50 years in the making, over which I have learned so much, been let down more often than not, betrayed, misguided and left disillusioned—inspired, loved, trusted, forgiven and supported. Throughout it all, the one thing that has always stayed constant is my work ethic, honesty, integrity, love of people and my belief that there is good in everyone, coupled with my burning desire to succeed.

When I started this book 20 years ago, I was your typical Aussie jock and aspired to motivate the masses through physical health. Yet, I have learned through my personal and professional journey that there is so much more to health and happiness. So, I am determined to share what I have learned to help minimise the risk for others and incentivise you to create change. This will allow you to reach your potential and ultimate happiness, hopefully with minimal personal/professional lows and many more highs.

I was raised in a stable family with two older sisters and loving parents who still have a great relationship. We grew up on the Mornington Peninsula in Mt Eliza, Victoria. Both Mum and Dad provided an extremely comfortable family environment.

My Dad was an accountant and worked for himself. He worked long hours to provide our family with the lifestyle offered to us. Long days, late nights and weekends. You name it, Dad did it, and he knew that it was all about making sacrifices to succeed. He didn't have an option; he was self-employed, had a large employee base and had three kids at private schools.

Mum worked even harder running the family, and now that I am a father of three, I am incredibly grateful for my childhood and the opportunities we were given. Towards the end of my schooling years, I remember discussing with Dad what life could look like after school as I was looking for direction. His advice was simple, but it has stuck with me: 'Tory, I don't care what you do, but whatever you do, be self-employed.'

Finding success in business: the journey to growth

So that is precisely what I did. After completing my university and postgraduate studies, I travelled and lived overseas for two years before starting my first business in February 2001. I started with a $20,000 loan from the bank, which allowed me to purchase some equipment to open a small mobile personal training company.

Over the next few years, my business continued to grow and evolve, with more staff and cars on the road. I offered personal training services in and around Melbourne. After three years, I developed my business significantly, and within four years, it had grown to become a national corporate health company, turning well over a million per annum.

Throughout my professional journey, I have experienced considerable personal and professional development throughout my core industry (health and fitness), not to mention the other businesses I have started, bought and sold, from a mobile juice company to a group training business and an online activewear company. I also founded and created an isotonic sports drink (that never made it to market) with a few mates. My most recent and career-defining business was investing heavily in not one, but two hospitality franchises. Unfortunately, the owner's talk was more extensive than their expertise, support and delivery.

Nevertheless, the lessons I have learnt as a business owner, father, husband and friend have been challenging and harder on my wife. You name it, we've experienced it together. The thrill of conquering mind over body, running 12 ultra marathons and completing 14 marathons. Finding love, getting married and bringing new humans into the world, having three beautiful kids, Indie, Tommy and Billy. Building wealth through health and working in the industry for over 20 years, then losing wealth in hospitality.

Navigating the tough times: learning resilience

Working for yourself is hard, but the only option is to keep working. Over my years in hospitality, I faced many challenges at home and work. I had limited resources to gain strength, get out of the grind and push through. I had to develop resilience to keep going; no other option appealed to me. I had to eliminate negative people. I had to stop negative thoughts. I just had to keep breathing, pushing day in and day out, hoping the tide would turn the next day.

At times, it felt like I was drowning; I could see the lifeguards, but they couldn't see me. It was incredibly lonely. The negative self-talk was soul-destroying, but I didn't like the alternative, so I only had one option: keep swimming!

I was angry, disappointed, embarrassed, ashamed and broken at worst. I kept reminding myself that my skillsets were my mental ability to disassociate and my physical health and fitness. I worked to provide my young family with a good lifestyle, only to tear it all up and invest in something I knew nothing about, believing it would bring me more time and money. How wrong I was!

Many people say money doesn't matter, so I challenge you to lose it all first and then ask that question again. You don't need millions of dollars, but we all need food, shelter and the ability to pay the bills. We all like security, and at least money gives you that.

Although the journey to exit hospitality was long and extremely challenging, I learned an important lesson. Stay strong and listen, but don't always act; trust yourself and never lose sight of your end goal, regardless of how bad it gets.

The easy option would have been to stop the grind, but is that the reward I sought? The one critical ingredient to gaining clarity is to dedicate time to yourself, for yourself. Speak to those you trust, care about and love. Ask yourself who's on your team and let the others listen to your voice message. You'll be able to count on one hand how many people are willing to help you. Conversations are one thing, but actions are the test, trust me!

Strength through adversity: finding clarity in tough moments

My journey taught me much about human behaviour, relationships, friendships, partnerships and personal resilience. *Blokes Inc. Play a Bigger Game* is much more than a self-help book to educate you on creating health and happiness. It's about giving you inspiration, strength and the confidence to keep pushing when circumstances are against you. It is about giving you the tools to design the life you want to lead. I will encourage you to embrace the grind, stay positive and trust yourself, as you are the only one who knows and understands what you want. Like all the best companies, sporting teams or organisations in the world, you will need a few elite team members in your corner to keep you accountable and provide structure, consistency and support.

Blokes Inc. Play a Bigger Game isn't here to teach you how to be a star athlete, the perfect partner or a top-notch parent. I won't tell you how to start a business, strike it rich, or give you tips on real estate or the stock market. I will offer you real education, inspiration and motivation—along with powerful stories from clients I've trained, coached and mentored. The tools I've developed and refined in *Blokes Inc. Play a Bigger Game* are about helping you create lasting change and achieve meaningful results.

Throughout the book, I focus on all facets of wellness, including mindset, nutrition, exercise, stress, sleep, social connectivity, sex and bio-individuality. If you have not heard of bio-individuality before, it means recognising that we are all unique and that achieving health and wellness is not a one-size-fits-all answer.

I am not going to pretend that life is not challenging and complex—but it can also be incredibly rewarding. The goal is to create more good days than bad and to stay well-rounded in all aspects of health and wellness.

Owning your path: consistency in wellness

Achieving wellness is about the basics: exercise, nutrition, sleep, hydration and social connection. Building these habits consistently creates the foundation of a multidimensional, healthy life. Simple routines, maintained consistently, are the most powerful tools for lasting change.

But first, a warning: change doesn't just happen. You must take ownership, trust your intrinsic motivation, and focus on your end goal. Keep your team close, and don't let roadblocks and failures define your end goal. Stay true to yourself. And ask yourself, if it's not you, then who?

I always tell my clients to treat their bodies like a business—you've got to stay on top of the details. Simple, consistent habits make the most significant difference. It's about stacking those habits and staying committed to the goal. That means having a solid exercise routine, eating natural, whole foods, staying hydrated, sticking to a consistent sleep schedule, and learning how to relax and stay socially connected. It's about becoming multidimensional and taking care of yourself in all areas.

After four years of darkness, how did I regain my clarity, reinvent my passion, improve my self-esteem and change my outlook?

Strength through adversity: finding clarity in tough moments

During my most challenging times, I leaned into what I knew best—investing in my physical and mental wellbeing. I focused on the present, letting go of regrets about the past and anxieties about the future. This journey taught me that health and happiness are built through daily commitment and perseverance, even when it is hard.

When I felt least able to keep going, I returned to what worked:

- I invested in my physical and emotional health.
- I stood up when I wanted to stay down.
- I found reasons to smile when I wanted to cry.
- I went to work, even on days when it cost more than it earned.
- I practised positive self-talk to drown out internal struggles.

I committed to leaving the past behind and setting aside endless worry about what was next. It is all about owning the present because right now is the only moment you can truly control. Believe that it is never too late to make meaningful changes if you are willing to make the daily effort for lasting progress.

Men often have an incredible appetite for competition, but when it comes to health and wellness, there is only one competitor: you. In isolation, you are the first dimension to fail. Having collaborated with people on their health journeys for over half my life, I have found it a fascinating experiment in human conditioning.

Many people are great talkers, but only a few are great doers. *Blokes Inc Play a Bigger Game* is about becoming a 'doer.' It's not about making excuses; it's about taking ownership of your lifestyle, understanding the direction you want to go and maintaining clarity.

Creating sustainable change: leveraging the core trio

Blokes Inc. Play a Bigger Game cannot provide a quick fix but can help you implement short-term solutions, like the core trio of what, how and when. These solutions will enable you to stay focused and committed to your vision, which will, in turn, determine your level of success.

Repeatedly, I tell people you don't go to bed with credit card debt and wake up a millionaire or go to bed obese and wake up buffed. *The Blokes Inc. Play a Bigger Game* journey is precisely that: a journey. There will be bumps and bruises; trust me, I've experienced them, but if you stay committed, stay strong, and, more importantly, stay focused and consistent, you can and will improve.

Life is challenging, filled with ups and downs and rarely gives us all the answers. Navigating relationships can feel like the world's most complex job, requiring patience, understanding and a willingness to grow, even when it is hard. Running a business on your own adds a unique layer of difficulty; self-employment can be a lonely journey full of doubts, long hours and the weight of every decision resting on your shoulders. And then, of course, there is the journey to staying healthy and happy—a path that is not always easy but brings the deepest rewards.

There is no magic recipe for success, but the formula itself is remarkably simple. It starts with one essential choice: you have the power to change. You can make the decision to show up, prioritise your wellbeing and put effort into meaningful connections. You can decide to work toward your dreams, no matter how many challenges appear. The real question is, are you willing? Are you prepared to push beyond your comfort zone and make those small daily commitments that build a multidimensional, fulfilling life?

Success, however you define it, does not come from just wanting change. It comes from a willingness to invest in yourself, to keep moving forward and to trust that each step brings you closer to the life you're capable of creating.

Redefining success: what really matters

For me, life is all about staying in the game for long enough to be good enough, and this starts with being honest with yourself.

Ask yourself what *you* want.

Is it the house, the fast car, the body, the bank balance, the pay rise, the job title, the sense of entitlement or the overseas holidays that define you? Or is it having a loving relationship, being a good partner, husband and father and being happy and healthy?

Whatever your goal and desire, it is 100% dependent on your commitment, consistency and control over your internal dialogue. Yet, if I can offer only one piece of advice, it would be to prioritise your physical and mental health because everything else is irrelevant without it.

I remember a great quote from the former chairperson and chief operating officer of Coca-Cola, Brain Dyson,

> *'Imagine life as a game in which you are juggling some five balls in the air…work, family, health, friends and spirit. You will soon understand that work is a rubber ball…but the other four are made of glass: family, health, friends and spirit.'*

Staying the course: trusting your vision

Blokes Inc. Play a Bigger Game is here to provide you with tools and inspiration for your journey. With honesty, self-awareness and dedication, I hope to equip you to pursue your vision and find fulfilment in every dimension of your life.

I will have succeeded in my goal if, through reading *Blokes Inc. Play a Bigger Game*, I pass on some of my education, enthusiasm and motivation, along with lessons from firsthand experiences, which will result in you reaching your personal and professional potential.

> *Live with purpose, play with passion, love with laughter.*
>
> —**Tory Trewhitt**

CHAPTER 2

Motivation, mindset and habits

Yesterday is history, tomorrow is a mystery, but today is a gift; that is why they call it 'the present.'

—Master Oogway (and others)

What it takes to achieve lasting wellness

This chapter explores what it takes to achieve lasting wellness: becoming multidimensional in both body and mind. Actual change starts with mastering your thoughts before your feelings because, without the right mindset, no amount of motivation will carry you through. The key is training your mind to embrace discomfort and keep pushing forward when tempted to retreat into your comfort zone.

The battle in your mind

Let's be honest: if getting fit and healthy were easy, we wouldn't be facing a global epidemic of lifestyle diseases, most of which are entirely preventable. The biggest battle lies in *the gap*—the space between your ears. If you can conquer your mind, you're already halfway to achieving optimal health and wellbeing. It won't be easy, but it will be your most rewarding journey. So, I challenge you to commit and embrace the process entirely.

When I initially entertained the concept of publishing a book to help motivate the masses, it was 100% focused on my career, personal brand and an opportunity to grow the business. At that stage, I was single, had no kids and thought it would be great exposure for my brand.

For one reason or another, it has since taken me 20 years to get the book on the shelf, but what I have gained, personally and professionally, now makes this book so much more authentic. I've tested my resilience, self-worth and wife's patience. I have experienced stress, financial hardship and many emotional battles as I have navigated through these experiences and poor (potentially unlucky) business decisions/ventures. I am also now 15 years happily married and have three kids. Our kids have seen and heard too much as we struggled through the hospitality experience. But if you were to ask me today: 'What is my biggest driver in life?' It would be my family. My wife and three kids are my most outstanding achievement and my most crucial motivator.

Winning the day—one step at a time

When the alarm goes off at 5 am, it is time to win the day and focus on the future with the end goal entrenched in my grey matter. Some days, I'd love to stay in bed or hit the snooze button, but I know that behaviour keeps me further from my goal. Doing uncomfortable things creates positive behaviours that develop habits—and habits form change.

I remember listening to the *Huberman Lab* podcast featuring David Goggins, one of the world's greatest motivators. In this podcast, Goggins talked about the inner dialogue he struggles with daily to achieve greatness.

I had thought Goggins was born motivated by this internal drive. He described himself as the lowest human on earth, with no talent and no ability to learn, but he made a choice. He used to ask himself, what was he willing to sacrifice? What was he willing to give up to achieve what he was after?

Finding your motivation and reframing your mindset

If you can't think of your immediate motivator, this chapter gives you some clarity or direction. While reading this chapter, consider your internal dialogue about your health, friends, family and self-worth. Think about your pain points and the struggles you are having. The cause and effect they are having on you and your limiting beliefs.

Ask yourself, are you happy? What would make you happy? What needs to change today? Do you have a short-term goal? What do you want from this book?

Becoming multidimensional for lasting change

Regardless of where you are now or where you would like to be, one critical ingredient to succeeding is becoming multidimensional and establishing good habits (nutrition, daily exercise, sleep hygiene, mindfulness, social connectivity). We know motivation won't last forever, but habits will.

In the quest for better health and optimal wellbeing, *Blokes Inc. Play a Bigger Game* recognises the critical role of motivation, mindset and habits in shaping your behaviour and choices. I passionately believe that without one of these elements, you cannot have the others, which makes these three powerful forces the fundamentals for achieving lasting change.

Blokes Inc. Play a Bigger Game recognises that maintaining good health requires not only external stimuli like nutrition and exercise but also a deeply rooted intrinsic motivator.

In this chapter, I will look into understanding motivation, identifying inherent motivation, creating a positive mindset and why cultivating a growth mindset is the key to your long-term success. I will challenge you to reframe, reprogram and re-boost your internal dialogue while providing practical insights and actionable steps to enhance your motivation to establish healthy habits that will last.

So, let's get started.

Understanding motivation

Motivation is the 'ignitor,' the initial driving force behind your actions fuelled by internal and external factors. Having been involved in the health and fitness industry for over 20 years, I have found that the motivational formula depends on the individual and the intensity of their desire, the reward value of their goal and their expectations.

Firstly, it is essential to understand whether the crucial driver is sustainable or realistic. This question will best help you succeed and focus during challenging times. When things seem like they aren't going as planned, the stronger your desire, the more likely you will achieve.

Motivation is not a one-size-fits-all concept. It is a profoundly personal and dynamic force shaped by your values and experiences. So, ask yourself what will get you out of bed when you would rather stay under the covers in the morning.

> Is it your family, health, job or financial situation?
>
> How do you feel emotionally when you wake up in the morning?
>
> Do you suffer from Mondayitis?
>
> Are you motivated and excited every morning for what the day might bring, or do you feel like you are on the merry-go-round doing the same thing day in and day out?

Gandhi was motivated to bring freedom to the people of India and his reward was to see this goal obtained by peaceful demonstration with the support of many people within his lifetime.

Nelson Mandela could not live in silence in his homeland of South Africa under apartheid and chose a life in prison rather than giving in to racism. His reward for his beliefs and the support of many people worldwide was to see the eventual abolition of apartheid, the freedom of his people and his independence.

Okay, our lives might not be destined for political greatness, but to create lasting change, you need a reward. As you read this chapter, think about what would motivate you today to jump out of bed tomorrow. What is your crucial motivator when times are tough, when you are tired, exhausted or face a day-to-day decision? Will your driving force be strong enough to help you make the correct decision? What is your dynamic force? In Chapter 1, I shared how many days I went to work, fully aware that I was losing money. I would turn on the lights at the restaurant and greet customers with a smile, knowing they were enjoying themselves while, inside, I was struggling. My motivation was to keep fighting for my family. I kept up this routine, day in and day out, for years.

Finding your intrinsic motivation

Sitting in thought is essential; reflecting on your dynamic force is personal. Determine what will motivate *you* to create change. The most challenging part is starting something new, breaking a bad habit or committing to making a change. Unfortunately, very few people are willing to commit or, more importantly, stay committed, so I have created an unadorned *Blokes Inc. Play a Bigger Game* formula.

First, we motivate, massage the mind and nourish our learned (sometimes forced) behaviours until they become habits. Once you have established these habits, you rely more on them because your habits become just that, habitual.

As the definition explains, motivation is being continually interested and having the desire and intensity to achieve a specific goal in life. One of the training philosophies I have always preached is 'constant commitment equals completion,' or my lifestyle philosophy, 'It's a journey of sacrifices, not a destination desire that creates change.'

The process of doing things daily accumulates into positive actions and change. The compound interest effect of running your body like a business involves doing the little things consistently. Paying off your mortgage isn't sexy, but over time, owning your home is. Doing little things daily, building wellness wealth and investing in yourself is all about playing the long game.

In the words of Steve Jobs:

> *I reached the pinnacle of success in the business world. However, aside from work, I have little joy. Lying on my sick bed and recalling my whole life, I realise that all the recognition and wealth that I took so much pride in have*

> *paled and become meaningless in the face of impending death. Material things lost can be found, but one thing that can never be found when it is lost is life.*

Initially, you might have trouble establishing your key motivational driver, which is 100% normal. Most people find motivation around three critical areas: health, career and relationships/family. Your initial intrinsic motivation might not inspire you to continue; it might just be the ignitor to get you started. But as Steve Jobs said, investing in you, the asset, is what matters.

The real causes of behaviour change: beyond aesthetics

People tend to look at their physical or aesthetic angle first to change their behaviour. They revert to their growing waistline, their lack of cardiovascular conditioning, and their deteriorating muscle tone, but is this an accurate indicator of what is going on, or are these aesthetic changes just a by-product of their environment?

I know when I was deep in the hospitality depression, I wasn't exercising; I was eating poorly and drinking to forget how bad the days were. I lacked energy and had no intrinsic motivation to exercise. I distanced myself from friends and family. I was struggling to control 'the gap.'

All of my physical and emotional side effects were a by-product of the toxic environment I was working in. Often, there is an external influence that affects several dimensions rather than specifically targeting one. This imbalance causes a shift in your mindset, which leads to a lack of personal commitment to yourself.

I'll start tomorrow.
I'll start next week.
Once this deal is done.
I'm travelling a lot.
Next quarter is my quarter.

These are all common excuses for delaying your start date. Be honest, be upfront, and respect your health. So, my question is, what are you willing to sacrifice to achieve your desired goal? Is money really that valuable? The key driver should be prioritising yourself primarily. Allocate time for self-love and create a wellness blueprint to suit your demands and desired outcomes.

In the journey towards optimal wellbeing, intrinsic motivation becomes the anchor to withstand the storms of doubt and difficulty. It transforms health pursuits from mere obligations to meaningful, fulfilling journeys.

Therefore, throughout *Blokes Inc. Play a Bigger Game,* I encourage you to identify your intrinsic motivation and use it as a beacon to light the path to lasting health and personal growth. My passion is to help you determine your inherent motivation and become multidimensional. It is the key to cultivating a sustainable, integrated approach to wellbeing that will stand the test of time.

Creating a positive mindset

As a parent, exercise physiologist, performance coach, personal trainer and mentor, I constantly try to educate and inspire people to become their 'best selves' through health and fitness. Motivation, mindset and habits are the three powerful forces shaping your behaviour in the quest for better health.

Like everything, many variables influence one's emotional and physical performance, such as sleep, nutrition, hydration, confidence, social connectivity and emotional stability. I find myself constantly challenged with how I can motivate people to push through their limits to improve their performance.

Nevertheless, once you consider all those variables, only one key ingredient directly correlates with one's personality and performance: positivity. The secret is to create a positive mindset that will outlast your level of motivation over time. While motivation can provide the initial spark for change, it is the formation of positive habits that sustain progress and long-term wellbeing. For many of you, it will be learning to eliminate the white noise, the battle with 'the gap,' teaching the art of positive self-talk and staying accountable, enabling you to reach your end goal.

Understanding that a positive mindset is the architect of change, shaping your attitudes, actions, and outcomes is essential. It is the cornerstone of sustained motivation. *Blokes Inc. Play a Bigger Game* advocates the importance of structure, accountability and consistency, which allows a positive environment to flourish. Motivation and mindset are intricately connected; you fuel your motivation by developing a positive attitude. It is only by maintaining this attitude, motivation and mindset that your success and wellbeing are achieved.

Why? Because attitude, motivation and mindset play a crucial role in shaping actions and outcomes. Motivation, a positive mindset and habit stacking give you an excellent chance of success.

All three are interconnected behaviours that complement each other. The importance of developing a positive mindset cannot be overstated in the context of motivation and performance success.

Blokes Inc. Play a Bigger Game champions the idea that a positive attitude is not only a precursor to motivation but also the driving force behind sustained effort, resilience and the realisation of personal and health-related goals.

The power of a growth mindset

The key to your continued success is understanding the concept of mindset and the two types: fixed and growth mindset. Let's dig deeper and look into these mindsets and how you can shift from one to the other.

As it states, a 'fixed' mindset is precisely that; it is characterised by the belief that our qualities, intelligence and abilities are traits that cannot be changed or improved. People in this state believe their talents and capabilities are predetermined and innate.

Unfortunately, their behaviours are often limited as they consider their abilities and actions cannot be changed, developed, improved or altered. This 'fixed' mindset determines their perceived limitations.

Whereas someone who believes their qualities, intelligence and abilities can be developed through effort, practice and learning is said to have a 'growth' mindset. They embrace challenges and opportunities, understanding that ability can be cultivated over time. This is the category I want you to harness.

Many of you might be pre-programmed to believe you are either one or the other; in *Blokes Inc. Play a Bigger Game*, I will challenge the fixed mindset and growth mindset dichotomy, asserting that mindsets can vary based on intentional effort and self-awareness. Mindset, often perceived as fixed, is a malleable force influenced by experiences.

Over my years as an educator and motivator, I have seen many people who believe they are either one or the other, typically brought upon by environmental factors. When others say, 'You can't do that,' 'That will never work,' or 'That doesn't suit your personality,' it 'fixes' the child's mind into a particular mindset.

It is essential to understand that you are not necessarily born with a fixed or growth mindset. Many influences shape how you function; typically, this occurs in your formative years by people who don't know they impact your long-term behaviour. Your social environment, upbringing, education and individual experiences are crucial to developing your mindset.

As mentioned above it is not predetermined at birth. You can and will change it if you desire to do so.

The power of action and intentional effort

My passion for authoring this book is changing behaviours, and the only way to do this is through action, intentional effort and self-awareness. Changing your mindset is no different.

Minimise the internal noise and the voices from the past questioning your qualities and abilities. Start with a sharp vision of what you want to achieve. Please write it down, take a picture, create a vision board and do whatever you can to shift your mindset and intentionally work to develop a growth mindset.

For a large part of my professional career, I have been motivating and mentoring individuals to shift their mindset, so now it is time for you to act and take ownership. No one else can do it for you; it must come from within your internal locus of control. Start by changing your attitude, leading to positive behaviours and actions and embracing the 'growth' mindset mentality.

Improve your success score by visualising the results you want. Journal about your experience and how it will feel when you achieve your end goal. Implement tools to increase your resilience, improve your motivation and help you overcome challenges.

Before moving on to the next chapter, try a few things and consider ways you could change your mindset by thinking more positively about behaviours and actions.

Creating and maintaining a positive mindset is imperative when changing behaviour. Your mindset can and will change based on the circumstances you face. You must understand this to implement strategies and tools to operate more often in a growth mindset and change your behaviour to achieve what you want.

Your mindset shapes your success

One of my favourite quotes is, 'Life is a game; you make the rules.' Your mindset plays a crucial role in shaping your experiences, your chosen actions and the happiness and success you achieve. A positive mindset, characterised by optimistic thinking, resilience and a growth-orientated attitude, can transform your life.

Unfortunately, getting fit, losing weight, paying off your credit card, saving for your dream house and developing a positive/growth mindset is not an overnight transformation but a continuous journey of self-discovery and personal growth. By recognising the power of your thoughts, embracing optimism and consciously reframing challenges, you can reshape your mindset and unlock your full potential.

> I have created a change model which includes three steps:
>
> 1. Motivation initiates change.
>
> 2. Consistency leads to change.
>
> 3. Habits sustain change.

Once you implement this model, your motivation becomes a learned behaviour. Then, you must cultivate habits and practices that will sustain your drive and enthusiasm over time. Through consistent effort and intentional actions, you can develop a mindset that naturally seeks motivation and finds fulfilment in pursuing your goals.

Nevertheless, it is essential to note that motivation may fluctuate naturally, even when it has become a learned behaviour, as many external factors influence this. The key to your level of success and ongoing motivation is establishing a solid foundation of learned behaviours and strategies that you can implement, which will proactively cultivate and reignite your level of motivation when required.

Let's dig deeper into learned behaviours.

How can you create learned behaviours?

In *Blokes Inc. Play a Bigger Game*, I highlight the importance of learned behaviours when boosting wellbeing. You can put several key strategies into practice—setting goals, building habits, becoming more self-aware, establishing routines, tracking your progress, staying accountable, adapting when needed and surrounding yourself with a supportive environment. If you implement these ideas, you'll be well on your way to maintaining long-term motivation and creating lasting, positive change.

There is no better way to start than by establishing a goal and creating an action plan to increase motivation and accountability. So, step one is identifying your end goal.

Then, break that goal into bite-sized pieces. Like the old saying, there is only one way to eat an elephant, one bite at a time. Creating several smaller, achievable goals along the way will develop a sense of progress and accomplishment, which adds fuel to your fire and leads to behaviours that complement your end goal.

Another step to creating continued learned behaviours is persistence, which enhances resilience and determination. Every setback becomes a chance to strengthen your ability to bounce back, allowing you to keep moving forward no matter the challenges. Resilience isn't about enduring—it's about growing stronger through each obstacle.

Nevertheless, changing behaviour becomes exceedingly difficult if you don't have a sense of self-awareness. Understanding your values, strengths and passion is essential, as is aligning your goals and actions accordingly and this is where the critical ingredients of accountability and adaptability are crucial. By leverageing your strengths, you can find greater meaning and intrinsic motivation and then, through self-reflection, you can honestly assess your progress. Then, if necessary, you can adjust your strategies to allow you to maintain your focus on your long-term goal.

This is one of the key reasons I encourage all my clients to identify a team of people who 'add' value to them. Returning to my analogy of running your body like a business, you need KPIs, you need to be challenged, you need to be supported, and you need to be kept accountable.

Therefore, to effectively use motivation to create behavioural change, it is crucial to employ strategies that cultivate and nurture it.

> To do this, you need three things:
>
> 1. You need to find out why. This is your intrinsic motivation and associates your values with behavioural change.
>
> 2. You need to understand your why. Ask yourself why it is essential for you to achieve your desired outcome.
>
> 3. You must set specific and meaningful goals aligned with the desired behavioural change.

The art and impact of habits

For many of you reading this book, your number one motivation might be to create change. There may be one area in your life you are not satisfied with. For some of you, your current behaviours might not align with or complement the healthy habits/behaviours required to create change.

Habits are behaviours performed automatically, reducing the reliance on conscious decision-making and willpower. Habits are learned behaviours that need to become long-lasting, recurring behaviours through consistency and a deliberate process of repetition.

> For many of you looking to change, building new habits is essential. The easiest way is to start with specific, achievable goals and then to follow these steps below to guide you to building healthy habits:

1. **Start small:** Begin with achievable, manageable changes. Small, gradual steps are more likely to become lasting habits.

4. **Set clear goals:** Define specific health goals to guide your habit-building process. Clear goals help motivate and focus your efforts.

5. **Establish a routine:** Consistency is critical. Incorporate your chosen health behaviours into a daily/weekly routine.

6. **Monitor progress:** Monitor your habits and their effects on your health. This provides accountability and feedback.

7. **Stay accountable:** Share your thoughts and goals and bring your support crew on your journey. External accountability can help you stay on track.

8. **Adapt and evolve:** Life is dynamic, so be prepared to adapt your habits to your circumstances and changes in your goals.

9. **Stay patient.** Habit-stacking takes time. Be patient with yourself and acknowledge that setbacks are all part of the process.

In *Blokes Inc. Play a Bigger Game*, I offer guidance to help individuals make lasting lifestyle changes by focusing on developing positive habits. I aim to help you initiate change and embed new behaviours into your daily life. If you can achieve this, you'll be well on your way to becoming a more multidimensional version of yourself.

Five-step blueprint to improve motivation, mindset and habits

Step 1: Define your why

Understanding your deeper purpose is the foundation of lasting motivation. Ask yourself why you want to make changes—whether for your health, family, career or personal growth. Reflect on your core values and the impact you want on your life and those around you. Keep this 'why' at the forefront of your journey to remind you when motivation wanes.

Step 2: Set clear, achievable goals

Start with small, realistic goals that are specific, measurable and time-bound. Break larger objectives into manageable steps to avoid feeling overwhelmed. For example, if improving fitness is a goal, start with a 20-minute daily walk instead of committing to an hour at the gym immediately. Celebrate each milestone to build momentum and confidence.

Step 3: Cultivate a positive mindset

Your mindset shapes your reality. Develop a growth mindset by embracing challenges, learning from setbacks and viewing effort as a path to mastery. Practice self-compassion and challenge negative self-talk by reframing setbacks as opportunities to learn. Surround yourself with positive influences and seek out mentors or community members who uplift and inspire you.

Step 4: Build consistent habits

Habits are the building blocks of a prosperous lifestyle. Focus on consistency over intensity. Start with one habit at a time, such as drinking more water, getting to bed earlier or dedicating 10 minutes daily to meditation. Use cues, such as setting reminders or creating routines, to help solidify these habits in your daily life. Remember, consistency beats perfection.

Step 5: Create a supportive environment

Your environment plays a crucial role in shaping your behaviours. Surround yourself with people who support your goals and remove obstacles that hinder progress. This might mean cleaning out your pantry, setting up a designated workout space or joining a community like *Blokes Inc. Play a Bigger Game* on social media where you can connect with others on the same journey. Accountability and a sense of belonging can significantly boost motivation and keep you on track.

By following these five steps, you'll be well on your way to improving your motivation, mindset and habits, setting the stage for a healthier, happier and more fulfilled life.

Remember, this is just the start and change takes time. Setbacks along the way are all part of the journey. The lessons you learn from the failed attempts will be the key to your long-term success. Just be patient with yourself and stay consistent.

What, how, when: the core trio for motivation, mindset and habits

1. What:

- Define your focus: Identify your goal to improve motivation, mindset and habits. This could be a personal goal, a shift in perspective or a habit you want to build.

- Motivation: *What* drives you? Is it better health, more energy or being a role model?

- Mindset: *What* beliefs or attitudes do you need to adopt? Perhaps resilience, positivity or a growth mindset.

- Habits: *What* actions will you take consistently? Daily exercise, mindful eating or regular sleep patterns.

2. How:

- Plan your approach: Determine how you will achieve your focus areas. This involves breaking down your goals into actionable steps and strategies that align with your lifestyle. Consider the resources, tools or support systems you'll need.

- Motivation: *How* will you stay motivated? Create vision boards, set up reminders of your 'why,' or track progress visually.

- Mindset: *How* will you cultivate the right mindset? Practice affirmations, mindfulness, journalling or seek feedback and learn from others.

- Habits: *How* will you implement new habits? Use habit stacking, start small and scale up, or set cues and rewards to reinforce behaviours.

3. When:

- Establish timing and consistency: Lastly, specify *when* you will act. Timing is crucial for building consistency and making your goals part of your routine. Schedule your actions into your daily or weekly calendar to ensure they happen.

- Motivation: *When* will you review your goals or reflect on progress? Set a specific time each week for self-reflection or planning.

- Mindset: *When* will you practice mindset shifts? For instance, begin each morning with gratitude or end each day with a reflection on what went well.

- Habits: *When* will you perform your new habits? Attach them to existing routines, like stretching after your morning coffee or meditating before bed.

Take the first step towards lasting wellbeing: create your personalised motivation, mindset and habits

Take control of your motivation, mindset and habits by focusing on the what, how and when. Doing so will create a clear and actionable formula that seamlessly integrates into your daily life. This approach helps you stay on track and empowers you to overcome obstacles, make consistent progress and achieve your goals with confidence and purpose. It is time to move beyond dreaming and implement the steps leading you to lasting success. Make it happen—starting now.

WRITE DOWN YOUR PLAN HERE:

What:
_____
_____
_____
_____
_____
_____
_____

How:
_____
_____
_____
_____
_____
_____
_____

When:
_____
_____
_____
_____
_____
_____
_____

CHAPTER 3

Nutrition and improving your energy

When diet is wrong, medicine is of no use. When diet is correct, medicine is of no need.

—Ayurvedic proverb

The pillars of lasting success

Several key themes emerge throughout this book, starting with the fundamental pillars for lasting success: sound nutrition, quality sleep and regular exercise. These wellness dimensions provide the foundation for building a successful, multidimensional plan.

Many people are driven by their emotions, which often influence their actions. Regarding nutrition, this emotional influence can be your biggest obstacle. That's why I encourage you to develop the ability to manage your emotions and shift your mindset to eat for purpose and performance, not just for pleasure.

In this chapter, I'll focus on educating and providing practical tools to help you control cravings and make more intentional food choices.

A real-life wake-up call: Andrew's story

Andrew, a 42-year-old professional, was deeply immersed in a high-stress career, earning a lot of money but putting his health at risk every day. His hectic lifestyle led him into poor eating habits, which were taking a serious toll on both his physical and mental wellbeing. He lived fast—up at 5 am, in bed by midnight, fuelled by caffeine in the morning and a couple of glasses of wine in the evening to unwind.

A typical day for Andrew involved grabbing a coffee before training, followed by another coffee on his commute. Breakfast was often something quick and carb-heavy, like a croissant or an egg-and-bacon muffin. Lunch was skipped, water was scarce and he kept his energy levels up with more caffeine and frequent trips to the office vending machine. Business dinners were typically washed down with plenty of alcohol. This routine—long hours, stress, junk food and alcohol—had become a habit and his way of coping with such a busy lifestyle.

Over time, this lifestyle started catching up with him. He gained weight, felt constantly fatigued and relied increasingly on caffeine, energy drinks and processed foods to get through the day. The dreaded

3 pm slump became routine and he'd combat it with yet another coffee or sugary soft drink. Despite his professional success, his health was spiralling.

The wake-up call came during a work trip to Sydney. Andrew, who regularly flew from Melbourne to Sydney for business, felt an unusual pain in his left calf, struggled to catch his breath and was hit with a pounding headache. As the plane ascended, sharp chest pain gripped him and he found it hard to breathe. Panicked, he hit the call button and flight attendants rushed to his aid who could see the passenger in distress. Within minutes, one of the flight attendants put the call through the cabin requesting any doctors or nurses to come to row 11. Luckily, a doctor appeared, assessed him and administered some oxygen. The initial diagnosis was a suspected a case of deep vein thrombosis (DVT), which was a condition often caused by prolonged periods of inactivity, which in Andrew's case was very accurate.

As the flight crew comforted the passenger an ambulance was requested to meet the plane when it landed in Sydney. Still to this day when Andrew reflects on this episode, he is embarrassed, but he also realised this was the turning point he needed. He'd always seen himself as invincible, but this health scare forced him to confront the reality of his choices. The 'important' business meeting he was flying to no longer seemed important. His unhealthy lifestyle had finally caught up with him and it was time for a change.

Implementing practical change: Andrew's journey

Fortunately, recognising the need for change, Andrew sought guidance from me, and the brief was to develop a tailored 'lifestyle' plan to accommodate his busy work schedule along with his travel commitments. The emphasis was on practicality and incorporating achievable changes yielding long-term benefits. I emphasised there was no quick fix, this needed to be a lifestyle change.

In the corporate sector, this is a common occurrence that I have dealt with day in and day out, but not usually after a DVT episode. The typical scenario is that an overweight, high achiever pays little attention to their health and wellbeing. They know what they should be doing but lack the structure to change and many aren't consistent enough for long enough.

So, for Andrew, accountability needed to be one of the key ingredients of his new program. Setting boundaries and creating structure around what he ate in the morning, on the commute and in the office. Together, we addressed the types of foods he was consuming, particularly the ratio between his macronutrients (carbohydrates, protein and fats), his portion sizes and the convenience of fast food/packaged foods.

When we commenced the accountability program, we made it clear that Andrew's requirements were to fill in a daily food diary, particularly looking at the time and type of food he consumed. Andrew also had to account for what he ate, the time of the day and the portion size. He also had to write down how he felt 20 minutes afterwards. With guidance, Andrew gradually transitioned from fast food binges to a balanced and nutrient-dense diet.

Organising for success: mindful food choices

One of the key behavioural changes that Andrew implemented was around his organisation and preparation. This created greater awareness when choosing the right food at airport lounges or when he was on the go. I spent time educating Andrew on the foods he could buy if he ate on the run. I taught Andrew how to read food labels so that if he understood what he was grabbing when reaching for that food bar or drink. Every item he bought over the counter, Andrew would know the energy value and the amount of sugar, fat and sodium rather than being swayed by the marketing hype on the package.

If Andrew was travelling, I knew his energy output would be low, so we had to adjust his eating options to accommodate his sedentary work environment. It was all designed around formulating a structured meal plan to suit Andrew's needs, considering work, travel, convenience, sustainability and exercise.

The lesson: health comes first

Andrew's mid-flight experience taught him a valuable lesson about the importance of self-care. He vowed never to let his health retake a backseat, knowing that a healthy body and mind were the keys to a fulfilling life.

Time to get real

With Andrew in mind as an example of how not to recognise whether your health is at risk, it is time to 'feel' the pain points. Start by looking, feeling and prodding your 'guts.'

> Look in the mirror and ask yourself:
> 1. How do I look?
> 2. How do I feel?
> 3. How are my energy levels?
> 4. How is my waistline?

Are you happy and content to join the 'dad-bod' community? No one judges you here, but if you want to lose a few kilos, take notes in this chapter and the one after it. Understanding the information is one thing, but the key to weight loss will be the implementation phase, putting your new knowledge into practice and sticking to the cause. The key to lasting changes is lifestyle changes and habit stacking.

In this chapter, I'm not drastically changing the way you eat; my focus will be educating you on the food groups you should eat. I will not get you to take a pill or get you to starve yourself for aesthetic purposes.

I will highlight the importance of eating 'real' foods and encourage you to double your water intake and consume more protein. Your food plan needs structure for lasting results. My focus will be on creating a healthy relationship with food and understanding that food is energy regardless of how healthy it is.

Real food: water consumption and protein intake

When it comes to your health and fitness, you can do so much right, but if you aren't fuelling your body correctly, you will not get the result you are after. You will become disillusioned and, more often than not, revert to your old habits.

There is an old saying that you can't out-train a bad diet. You can run, jump, swim, push, meditate, plunge and much more, but you must eat the right foods to gain, lose or maintain weight. In the fast-paced world we live in today, peak performance, whether it's on the athletic field, in the classroom, the boardroom or in the bedroom, one fundamental aspect that often takes centre stage is nutrition. The food we consume is the cornerstone of our physical and mental capabilities, influencing our energy levels, cognitive function, mood and overall wellbeing.

We must invest in our long-term health and vitality by making conscious, nutritious choices and embracing various foods. I respect that the journey to improving your nutritional platform is a personal one that continually evolves. For me, it's not about perfection; it's about progression.

Trust me, my diet isn't perfect. As you work through this chapter, it's important to remember that food is a medicine; embrace it with an open mind, create small changes, savour the flavours and allow it to become an integral part of your life's journey toward better health.

I want to educate you on the importance of food. I want you to understand that food can and will either 'hurt' or 'heal' you. I also want to give you the knowledge to make the right choices. During this chapter, I will highlight the pivotal role nutrition plays in achieving and sustaining optimal performance, which is the purpose of this book.

A good nutritional plan is the cornerstone of feeling and functioning well, impacting every aspect of your physical and mental health. Like a grand symphony, I liken healthy eating to a beautifully orchestrated piece of music where each food group plays a crucial role.

When we include all food groups, or macronutrients, in our diet, our body experiences energetic crescendos for our daily performance. Just like the pipes of a grand organ, our body's systems align and function optimally, leading to a harmonious existence. Nourishing food is the conductor of this symphony, orchestrating a balance that influences our physical vitality, cognitive clarity and overall wellbeing. Proteins, carbohydrates, fats, vitamins and minerals contribute to this symphony, ensuring that our body and mind are well-nourished and in tune.

When we neglect quality food groups or consume an imbalanced diet, the chorus of our body's functions risks failing. Without the proper nutrients, our energy levels plummet, our cognitive function suffers, and our overall health deteriorates. I encourage you to become the 'conductor.' Just as a symphony requires the careful arrangement of different musical elements, a good diet requires the mindful inclusion of various food groups. By nourishing our bodies with a balanced diet, we can ensure that our life's symphony plays harmoniously, leading to better health and wellbeing.

Over the last decade or more, our relationship with food has changed dramatically. Our society has come to expect that everything is on demand.

Food holds tremendous power in shaping how we look, feel and function and plays a considerable part in our longevity. No longer are we influenced by seasonal food, which positively impacts our health. People are influenced by marketing companies and social media influences, which affect what, when and why they consume certain foods. We have become 'emotional eaters' not 'educated consumers.'

Progress, not perfection: building healthy eating habits

I acknowledge, respect and remember that nutrition is more than just fuel for your body; it's the raw material your cells need to function correctly. Simple sacrifices or changes can be made to your eating habits, but you must start now. Not after your holiday, the long weekend, the business trip or the party, as typically, you will always find an excuse. I get it and I fight it just as much as you. Saying no to cocktail food at parties, refusing leftover food from the kids and avoiding the temptation to buy something sweet when paying for petrol are easy habits you can install for better health.

Quitting the late-night fast-food stops after a few beers or refusing the food at sporting venues takes discipline, and discipline requires willpower. I encourage you to be brave enough and strong enough for long enough to allow these temptations to pass. Before you eat, ask yourself a simple question: Does this particular food group or snack *add* value, or are you just eating to fulfil your emotional hunger?

Like anything you want to change, the key to improving is creating a positive habit around your desired pain point. For the new, positive habit to be successful, the critical ingredient is consistency, which you can achieve through discipline.

ACTIVITY

ASSESS YOUR EATING HABITS

To improve your eating habits, start by understanding and educating yourself on the following:

- What food groups do you consume (carbohydrates, proteins, fats)?
  _____
- Understand your portion sizes.
  _____
- Are you consciously aware of how much water you consume daily?
  _____

I ask because you need to be able to answer these questions if you want to gain weight (muscle), lose weight (weight loss), or feel better about yourself and have more energy.

Everything takes time and the key is consistency.

ANSWER THE FOLLOWING:

- Do you regularly eat breakfast?
  _____
- Do you have healthy snacks during the day?
  _____
- Do you consume fruit and vegetables daily?
  _____
- Do you drink two or more litres of water a day?
  _____
- Do you know which foods are rich in carbohydrates, protein and fats?
  _____
- Do you know the difference between good fats and bad fats?
  _____
- Do you have an estimate of your calorie intake?
  _____

Well done if you answered 'yes' to all these questions; if so, you should fast-track to the 'calories' section in Chapter 4.

If you can't answer 'yes' to all of these questions, read on and ask yourself the same questions at the end of the chapter. Remember, when discussing the quality of your life and looking at ways to increase your health, respect that poor nutrition can and will kill you. Sure, it might be boring, but you need to invest in your health now to gain success later! As Hippocrates was alleged to have said: 'Let thy food be thy medicine and medicine be thy food.'

What is healthy eating

When we refer to healthy eating, the key ingredient is a variety of foods to promote overall wellbeing, support good health and reduce the likelihood of chronic disease. Unfortunately, this is one area where marketing companies continue to persuade our choices. 'Fat-free,' 'low fat,' 'no carbs,' 'sugar-free' and 'protein rich' marketing slogans all influence our food choices.

Healthy eating is about conscious choices in what you eat, when, and how you prepare your meals. The biggest mistakes people make are eliminating food groups, food selection/food quality (seasonal eating), and portion distortion (meal sizes). Healthy eating is not about strict dieting or deprivation but establishing sustainable, positive eating habits that last.

Remember, your eating plan needs to suit your environment, challenges, pain points, goals and function. Looking at Andrew, who we met earlier, we identified that after work or while commuting, he struggled with meal selection and alcohol consumption. Mornings were rushed and fuelled with caffeine and carbohydrates, while evenings were airport lounges or Uber Eats.

Another mistake many people make is that they fuel their taste buds, not their hunger and eat for the sake of eating. I'm 100% guilty of this, particularly when filling my car up with petrol. I occasionally grab the

Allen's Party Mix packet and then wrestle with myself not to finish the packet before I get home.

Many of my clients struggle with the finger food at social events or business functions because it is offered to them, not because they are hungry. A little self-control and organisation will make a massive difference to your nutritional plan and eating habits, and you will also notice improved physiological effects. You will have more energy, your concentration levels will improve, your sleeping patterns will improve, and your headaches will disappear.

Sound good? Then why don't you make a few simple modifications to your current eating habits? You might not feel better immediately, but you will feel better if you continually pay attention to your nutritional consumption; just ask Andrew.

What is a healthy food plan?

A healthy food plan is a bit like success; it differs for everyone. So, what does a healthy food plan look like for you? Consider what you can improve (food groups, meal sizes, hydration), keeping in mind that whatever choices you make must be sustainable. I would instead implement a lifestyle solution, not a short-term, quick fix that focuses on creating rapid weight loss.

> When addressing your food plan consider the following factors, your:
> - meal frequency
> - macronutrient distribution (carbohydrates, protein and fats)
> - hydration platform
> - emotional eating triggers
> - processed food intake.

Many people get confused when considering their nutritional habits, as the power of the marketing dollar often influences one's choices. Nevertheless, there are essential nutrients that you should include in your daily nutritional plan, which establish the framework of your meals.

These macronutrients are: carbohydrates, proteins, fats and essential vitamins and minerals. They are the building blocks of our cells, organs and body and the brains primary energy sources. All these food groups are necessary for optimal functioning, maintenance and repair, which is why, in modern society, fashionable diets that eliminate food groups are inadequate.

Let's discuss the three main macronutrients you should consume daily and include in your healthy food plan.

Carbohydrates

Sure, beer has plenty of carbohydrates, but that is not the way I encourage you to attain your recommended daily allowance. Carbohydrates are the body's primary and the brain's primary energy sources. You would be familiar with many types of carbohydrates, such as grains, legumes, fruits and starchy vegetables. Nevertheless, it is essential to familiarise yourself with both simple and complex carbohydrates.

Too many 'simple' carbohydrates will lead to tightening your pants or excess weight gain. Perhaps, even the bragging rights of a well-earned 'beer gut,' but secretly behind closed doors, you would like it to be gone.

So, while reading this chapter, start reviewing your eating habits, consider your carbohydrate consumption, break it down to simple versus complex carbohydrates and ask yourself what you could reduce, eliminate or change.

Simple carbohydrates

Simple carbohydrates are made of units or molecules of sugar and, in most cases, are sweet. They are the quick fixes you crave mid-afternoon, the foods in vending machines and often at checkouts.

Simple carbohydrates are the sugars that come from fruits, some vegetables, milk, sucrose or table sugar (from cane and sugar beet). Sucrose is added to ice cream, biscuits, chocolate, cakes and most carbonated soft drinks. These simple carbohydrates are a trap as they provide quick-release energy, meaning your body can break them down quickly unless you consume too many. So, when restructuring your healthy food plan, reduce the number of simple carbohydrates as these tend to be empty calories, in that they don't offer much nutritional value at all.

Complex carbohydrates

Complex carbohydrates contain dietary fibre and starches, which take longer to digest. This slower digestion helps regulate blood sugar levels, providing sustained energy and supporting overall health. Many complex carbohydrates, particularly those high in fibre, release energy gradually.

Complex carbohydrates are often found in whole foods like wholemeal bread, brown rice, whole grains, vegetables, and pulses. These are generally recommended over refined or 'white' carbohydrates, such as white bread, pasta, and rice, which contain less fibre and may cause quicker spikes in blood sugar and insulin levels.

Switching to wholegrain or wholemeal alternatives can be a straightforward way to improve your diet, as these options are higher in fibre, vitamins and minerals. Foods with a lower glycaemic value tend to support steadier blood sugar levels, which can be beneficial for weight management and metabolic health.

In contrast, refined carbohydrates (such as white bread and pasta) are digested more quickly, which can lead to faster rises in blood sugar and insulin levels. While managing blood sugar and insulin can support weight loss, a balanced diet combined with regular physical activity is essential, as exercise alone cannot offset the effects of a consistently poor diet.

Protein

Proteins are large molecules made up of amino acids. There are 20 different amino acids, of which nine are essential (meaning the body cannot synthesise them and they must be obtained through diet). These essential amino acids are critical for many biological processes, such as building tissues, enzymes and hormones. If you look at the properties of the human body and eliminate the amount of water, 50% of your weight is a protein source (Bruce et al. 2017).

Proteins are essential building blocks for muscles, skin, bones, hair and nearly every other body part or tissue. Despite its crucial role, protein's importance in the body is often overlooked. Proteins make up enzymes that drive chemical reactions, including haemoglobin, which carries oxygen in the blood.

Protein-rich foods are essential for the body's growth and repair, so you must understand which foods contain protein and address your eating habits to ensure adequate intake. Suppose you look at the recommended daily intake (RDI) for protein. In those guidelines, there are a few variables (age, gender and activity level), but I guarantee the majority of you still aren't consuming anywhere near enough protein daily. The RDI guideline typically is 0.8 g of protein per kilogram of body weight daily. I often advise clients to consume between 1.5–2.0 g/kg of body weight (*Harvard Health* 2015).

When reviewing your daily intake, consider the food groups you consume, as our society often overeats carbohydrates and under-consumes protein. An example of this is having cereal for breakfast, a sandwich for lunch and then pasta, rice and potatoes for dinner with a few vegetables and some animal protein. Most of the meal options that people consume frequently are predominantly carbohydrates.

Therefore, it is essential to restructure your meals so that you are at least trying to get 40 g of protein for each meal. To do this, you need to understand which foods are high in protein and then try to consume these foods first.

Omnivores have an easier time consuming 'complete' protein containing all nine essential amino acids since they eat various foods, including meat, fish, poultry, vegetables, fruits, grains and other plant-based foods. Vegetarians, especially vegans, may struggle to get enough complete proteins because they rely more on plant-based foods, which typically do not provide all essential amino acids in a single source. For example, to obtain complete proteins, plant-based eaters must combine foods—like chickpeas and lentils or grains and seeds—to cover the full amino acid profile.

While there are benefits to both animal and plant-based proteins, animal proteins naturally contain all nine essential amino acids, making them 'complete' protein sources. Plant-based proteins, on the other hand, are generally lower in saturated fats and cholesterol, which can benefit cardiovascular health. If you follow a vegetarian or vegan diet, combining various plant-based protein sources is crucial to ensure you get a complete amino acid profile. For a balanced intake, options like legumes, grains and seeds are ideal.

Ultimately, the goal is to ensure you get enough protein for optimal health, regardless of your diet. From a practical standpoint, let's consider Andrew again, who is out for dinner, and there is a six-ounce Porterhouse steak on the menu, just under 200 g; it is an excellent source of protein, packing 38 g worth. It also delivers 44 g of fat, of which 16 g are saturated fat.

The alternative for Andrew is to choose some salmon, which would give you the equivalent amount of protein, 34 g, with only 18 g of fat, of which only 4 g are saturated. The message here is that even though Andrew is making a relatively healthy choice in the steak, it is important to be consciously aware of the percentage of saturated fats accompanying some high-protein meal options.

Are you unsure of what animal to select when eating out, as you are consciously concerned about protein versus fat intake? Typically, I advise clients to choose the fastest (leanest) animal, fish or poultry.

Why do I put so much emphasis on protein? The simple facts are that if you don't consume enough protein, your body is at risk of muscle atrophy, decreased immunity, impaired growth and development, hormonal imbalances and nutrient deficiencies (Martone et al 2017). Protein-rich foods also provide essential vitamins, minerals and micronutrients. Insufficient protein intake may lead to deficiencies in other nutrients, such as iron, zinc, Vitamin B12 and Vitamin D.

Like Andrew, a 'typical' office worker who is sedentary, if he were to consume too much protein, this could also be detrimental due to the effect of gluconeogenesis, which is when glucose is produced from non-carbohydrate sources and typically elevates blood sugar levels. This can be easily averted through movement. Numerous studies have shown that going for a brisk walk post-meal is enough to stabilise your blood sugar level and stop you from going into a 'couch coma.'

High-protein food to include in your diet

Below is a list of high-protein food options you could include or substitute for your existing meal options. If you want a dietary overhaul, seek advice from a qualified professional.

Breakfast

High protein breakfasts could include:

- Greek yoghurt (preferably plain, unsweetened)
- eggs
- protein smoothie (I love a protein powder smoothie in the morning, ideally without fruit, as it will spike your blood sugar levels. If you are vegan, ensure your protein powder is pea and rice protein powder so that it is a 'complete' protein source.)
- cottage cheese (with nuts and berries or a slice of sour dough).

Lunch

High protein lunches could include:

- animal-based protein source (chicken, fish, turkey) in a salad wrap
- omelettes
- lentils with a salad or in stew/soup
- quinoa as a nutritious base for salads or grain bowls.

Dinner

High protein dinners could include:

- salmon, lean beef or chicken (add vegetables, rice or sweet potatoes)
- tofu or tempeh.

Snack options

High protein snacks could include:

- nuts and seeds
- protein bars/shakes (Bars 10 g protein but minimal sugar. Shakes 30 g protein per serving)
- jerky
- eggs
- yoghurt
- tofu.

So, start by understanding food types, which will allow you to then assess which you could include/substitute and which foods you should minimise. Make simple adjustments, such as increasing protein options, reducing highly processed carbohydrate intake daily, and including more meal planning and structure around your meals.

A simple rule I get clients to incorporate is that when they are eating out, they should eat the protein on their plate first, then their vegetables or salad, and then the starchy carbohydrates if they can still fit it in.

Another essential food group that always provokes negative thoughts is fats. So, let's review fats and understand why they are necessary to consume and the difference between the 'good' and the 'bad' fats.

Fats

From media reports to marketing campaigns, through to the neighbour next door, people are obsessed with fat. People are obsessed with eating fat, getting fat and/or losing fat. Whatever the fat is, everyone is talking or thinking about it, yet it has similar considerations to carbohydrates: there are 'good' and 'bad' fats.

It is worth understanding that fats play a crucial role in establishing healthy eating habits and are an essential nutrient for optimal health. Firstly, fats are a concentrated energy source, providing essential fatty acids that the body cannot produce alone. These fatty acids are crucial for brain health (cognitive function), hormone production and cell function. Fats also slow digestion, helping you feel fuller for longer and reducing the likelihood of overeating. So, when designing a healthy eating plan, don't fear the word 'fat;' instead educate yourself and understand the difference between 'good' and 'bad' fats.

Good fats

Good fats, also known as healthy fats, promote overall health and wellbeing. Good fats are essential to the body because they assist in both energy production and strengthen the immune system. They also speed up the metabolism, assist the body in transporting vitamins, help purify the blood and help fight against disease, cancer, arthritis and other joint problems.

We don't always have to have negative connotations with the word 'fat.' Consuming 'good' fats is done in the form of unsaturated fats, monounsaturated oils and fats and polyunsaturated fats. These fats can be found in foods like avocados, nuts, seeds and fatty fish, like salmon and mackerel.

When you want to consume good fats or choose a dressing, a pasta sauce, or a dish at a restaurant, look at the ingredients (or ask the waitperson) for olive oil, nuts, eggs, linseed oil and sunflower seeds. More often than not when you are eating out, the fat in the dressing or the sauce causes the weight gain, not the protein source on your plate. These fats are classified as 'bad' (saturated/trans fats) and should be consumed in moderation.

Bad fats

To maintain a healthy diet, it's important to limit or avoid consuming 'bad' fats, known as saturated fats, which offer little to no nutritional benefit. These fats are commonly found in processed foods like fatty meats, butter, margarine, cheese and pastries. Saturated fats can negatively affect your health by raising your low-density lipoprotein (LDL) or 'bad' cholesterol, which can increase blood pressure. Over time, this can cause your blood to thicken and lead to fatty deposits inside your arteries, increasing the risk of a heart attack in severe cases.

Eating a diet high in saturated fats increases the risk of thicker blood, higher blood pressure, a slower metabolism, and lifestyle-related diseases like weight gain, chronic inflammation, reduced insulin sensitivity and cardiovascular disease—and who wants that? Some research has suggested that a high intake of fat, particularly trans fats, may be linked to an increased risk of cognitive decline, Alzheimer's disease and other neurological disorders (Malik et al 2024).

Take a moment to consider your nutritional intake. Are you consuming too much saturated and trans fats? These fats are found in many processed and fried foods, including fast food, packaged snacks, baked goods and margarine. That's why I encourage you to avoid late-night fast-food cravings and stay clear of the work vending machines. The key is to look at your current meal/snacking options and how to reduce your intake of 'bad' fats and focus on consuming 'good' fats. The best way to do this is by choosing lean protein sources, opting for low-fat or fat-free dairy products, minimising packaged foods, cakes, biscuits and creamy sauces and limiting the amount of processed and fried foods you consume.

COMPARISON OF 'GOOD FATS' AND 'BAD FATS' MEAL OPTIONS

GOOD FATS MEAL OPTIONS	BAD FATS MEAL OPTIONS
Avocado and poached or scrambled eggs on whole grain toast.	**Burgers:** any fast-food burger is typically high in saturated fat, combined with processed cheese and a white flour bun.
Salmon salad: mixed greens topped with grilled salmon, avocado slices and dressing with olive oil and lemon juice.	**Hot chips** are great for a hangover but have little nutritional value. Due to the frying process, they are also high in 'bad' fats.
Greek yoghurt parfait: Greek yoghurt layered with mixed berries and nuts, drizzled with honey.	**Pastries:** most bakery products harm your waistline. Croissants and doughnuts are high in trans fats and saturated fats due to the butter or shortening used in the baking.
Grilled chicken and veggies: grilled chicken breast served with a side of roasted vegetables.	**Creamy alfredo pasta:** high in saturated fat from the cheese and cream.
Quinoa and black bean bowl: quinoa, black beans, avocado, corn, tomatoes and a squeeze of lime juice.	**Any fried food:** more often than not, deep fried food contain trans fats from the frying oil (invest in an air fryer).

Do you remember what I mentioned at the start of this chapter: all food groups have an energy value; regardless of how healthy it is, everything contains calories. It doesn't matter how good your nutritional platform is, you will gain weight if you consume more calories than you use.

So, in Chapter 4, let us improve your eating habits. Then, in Chapter 5, we can address your exercise habits, a crucial part of your health improvement journey. Combining a sound nutritional plan and a regular exercise routine will hopefully motivate you and improve your overall health and vitality.

Curating your nutritional blueprint

Before you compile your nutritional blueprint, let's explore a few nutrient-dense foods that provide a high concentration of essential nutrients relative to their calorie content. These types of food are rich in vitamins, minerals and antioxidants. The easiest way is to consume various nutrient-dense foods from varying macronutrients.

NUTRIENT-DENSE FOODS TYPES

FOOD	TYPE
Leafy greens	Spinach, kale and collard greens contain Vitamins A, C and K, minerals like iron and calcium, antioxidants and fibre.
Vegetables	Broccoli, cauliflower, Brussels sprouts, and cabbage are excellent sources of Vitamins C and K, folate, fibre and phytonutrients.
Berries	Blueberries, strawberries, raspberries and blackberries are rich in vitamins, antioxidants and fibre.
Fish	Fatty fish, like salmon, mackerel and sardines, provide omega-3 fatty acids essential for heart and brain health.
Nuts and seeds	Almonds, walnuts, chai seeds and flaxseeds are packed with healthy fats, protein and various vitamins and minerals.

Eggs	Eggs are a reliable source of protein, Vitamin B12, choline and other essential nutrients.
Legumes	Beans, lentils, chickpeas and peas are rich in protein, fibre, iron and folate.
Sweet potatoes	Sweet potatoes are loaded with Vitamins A and C, potassium and fibre.
Greek yoghurt	Greek yoghurt is high in protein, calcium and probiotics that support gut health.
Quinoa	Quinoa, a nutrient-rich grain, provides protein, fibre, magnesium and various vitamins.
Avocado	Avocados are a great source of monounsaturated fats, potassium, vitamins E, K and C.
Tomatoes	Tomatoes are rich in Vitamin C, potassium and the antioxidant lycopene.
Oranges	Oranges are known for their Vitamin C content and other vitamins and minerals.
Lean meats	Lean chicken, turkey and lean beef cuts provide high-quality protein and essential nutrients like iron and zinc.
Mushrooms	Mushrooms are a source of B vitamins, selenium and other essential nutrients.
Bell peppers	Bell peppers or capsicums as they are also known contain high levels of vitamins A and C, as well as antioxidants.
Seaweed	Seaweed is rich in iodine, minerals and antioxidants, especially in varieties like nori and wakame.
Asparagus	Asparagus are a great source of vitamins A, C, E and K, as well as folate and fibre.
Pumpkin	Pumpkins are rich in beta-carotene, fibre and antioxidants.

Customising your nutritional blueprint

Later, in Chapter 11, I will go into more detail about the concept of 'bio-individuality,' in relation to my clients as they typically look for that 'quick fix,' particularly in how they look, feel and function. Unfortunately, when it comes to nutrition, many people are making incorrect choices mainly because of generalised marketing messages.

I am passionate about people and education. Hopefully, by reading this chapter, you have gained enough knowledge to make the right choices when designing a nutritional blueprint to suit your goals, lifestyle, dietary requirements and preferences. Remember, everything in moderation is fine. Rather than reverting to the easy option, play the long game and stay consistent.

Tips to help you design your blueprint

Building a sustainable health plan starts with identifying your unique goals—whether it is gaining muscle, losing weight, or improving fitness and sleep. From there, focus on optimising your macronutrient intake, portion sizes and food choices to suit your lifestyle. Incorporating mindful eating, smart snacking and regular meal prep helps create a balanced, consistent approach. Supplements can enhance your progress if needed and above all, remember that consistency, not perfection, is the key to lasting results.

> Complete the following steps to design your blueprint:
>
> 1. Start by identifying what your individual goals are:
>   a. Increase muscle mass.
>   b. Decrease your weight.
>   c. Improve your fitness level.
>   d. Improve your sleeping habits.
>   e. Improve your athletic development.
>   f. Reduce your risk profile.

2. Think about your current macronutrient consumption and how you will improve it.

3. Consider your dietary preferences (vegetarian, vegan, omnivore) and any particular food tolerances.

4. Identify your food choices (fat, protein, carbohydrates) and address portion sizes.

5. Plan how you can incorporate food preparation into your weekly routine.

6. The art of snacking and thinking about what you currently snack on versus what you should snack on.

7. Plan how you will incorporate mindful eating into your day. Noticing how you feel before, during and after eating fosters a better connection with foods and prevents emotional or binge eating.

8. Supplements can be a welcome addition to your blueprint. Based on your blood test results and eating plan, assess whether you need extra supplements.

9. Finally, make sure your blueprint is sustainable. It is no good being fantastic for four weeks; consistency is the key to lasting results. Short-term behaviours equal short-term results. One bad meal won't make you fat, but many bad meals will.

ACTIVITY

DESIGNING YOUR BLUEPRINT (SAMPLE DAY BELOW)

Day/meal	Breakfast	Snack	Lunch	Snack	Dinner	Other
Mon	poached eggs sourdough bread ½ an avocado	egg muffin	chicken salad	protein shake	salmon fillet (150 g = 30g protein) roasted broccolini 1 cup brown rice	Snack options: Greek yoghurt protein balls unsalted nuts

HYDRATION EXAMPLE

Time	Drink	Amount
6 am	espresso	1 cup
7 am	water	½ glass
8 am	water	½ glass
9 am	medium latte	1 cup
10 am	nil	nil
11 am	nil	nil
12 noon	water	1 glass

Now, design your weekly eating and hydration blueprint:

MEALS

Day/meal	Breakfast	Snack	Lunch	Snack	Dinner	Other
Sunday						
Monday						
Tuesday						
Wednesday						
Thursday						
Friday						
Saturday						

HYDRATION DAILY SCHEDULE

Time	Drink	Amount

CHAPTER 4

Mastering nutrition: key principles for a balanced diet

> *Good nutrition is a responsibility, not a restriction.*
>
> —Betty Faust

The power of knowledge in nutrition

In this chapter, I will discuss calories and explain the art of reading food labels, portion distortion, fasting and fads. Education, although important, is only one component of your healthy eating plan. Implementing education is the key ingredient (pardon the pun) to creating change.

Remember the old saying that knowledge is power? Regarding your nutritional framework, knowledge is your energy through correct implementation. This challenging phase involves addressing your macronutrients, calorie intake versus expenditure, food quality and portion sizes. So, before you set about overhauling your nutritional habits, take some time to review the fundamental principles of healthy eating below.

> **Case study: Andrew's nutritional transformation**
>
> Let us return to my client, Andrew, to see the fundamental principles in action.
>
> When I started working with Andrew, his automatic response to hunger or thirst was heading to the vending machine. Therefore, my first goal for Andrew was to develop a structure for his eating. I focused on getting Andrew to introduce more whole foods to his diet and developing the habit of eating protein first, I encouraged him to stop grabbing muffins and I got him to swap the post-training coffee with a protein shake.

Creating a structured eating routine

One of the critical components to stopping Andrew from eating for pleasure was ensuring he had access to healthy snack options (boiled eggs, nuts, fruit, yoghurt, shakes). Typically, his afternoon snack was an emotional action.

Over time, we found that supplementation benefited Andrew by killing two birds with one stone. It improved his hydration, as well as his protein intake. I also ensured that his office incorporated fruits and vegetables and some hummus for snacks rather than packaged foods, chips and chocolate bars, which were his regular choices in the past.

Setting nutritional boundaries

Andrew's nutritional roadmap moving forward was based on the following:

- organisation and preparation
- structure
- mindfulness around meals
- meal consistency.

These four nutritional boundaries became integral to Andrew's daily routine and formed his food framework. Reflect on your nutritional framework and ask whether you eat specific foods for pleasure or performance.

From 6 am–6 pm, Andrew could easily manage his food choices, but he struggled outside his working hours, so we needed more structure and easy options to minimise any temptations at home. One initiative we implemented was a meal delivery service just for evening meals if he wasn't out with clients. Another positive about Andrew's meal delivery service was that it helped Andrew with his portion sizes and guaranteed he consumed adequate protein.

Over time, Andrew also overcame his reluctance to meal prep, ensuring that nutritious options were readily available when he got home from work: nuts, avocado, hummus, cottage cheese—simple high-protein snacks. Rather than grabbing a packet of chips, a chocolate bar and a can of coke at the closest petrol station.

The impact of small, consistent changes

Within a few months, the transformation was palpable. Once Andrew started experiencing increased energy levels, improved mood and a notable weight reduction, it was easy to eliminate the glass of red wine and the ham-cheese toasty at the airport lounge. I also deleted Uber Eats from his phone to minimise convenience.

Combining a healthier nutritional platform and newfound energy motivated Andrew to reintegrate exercise into his routine outside our training sessions, further boosting his physical and mental wellbeing. It was interesting that Andrew wanted to eat cleaner, drink more water, minimise emotional eating and exercise more once he started feeling better.

Within six weeks Andrew had more energy and started looking better, highlighting a personalised meal plan's significant impact on one's overall health and vitality. He had even dropped seven kilos, which was a bonus as it wasn't our initial focus.

The most challenging yet most straightforward step to fix initially was for Andrew to acknowledge the consequences of his current sedentary lifestyle, poor nutritional habits, and stressful job and their direct effect on his health. Andrew not only reversed the adverse side effects on his body (weight gain, lethargy, stress) from eating poorly and having no consistent exercise routine, but he also revitalised his mental and emotional wellbeing.

Consistency: the key to long-term success

This revitalisation didn't require a pill or a potion. It was just the consistency of healthy meal options and knowledge of food options. Andrew's simple formula was creating structure and implementing boundaries between 6 am and 8 pm. Outlining what he could and couldn't eat and drink, we focused on changing his relationship with food and respecting it as fuel for performance, not to satisfy hunger, fatigue or dehydration.

Key principles of healthy eating

The key principles of a healthy diet are:

1. **Balanced diet:** A healthy diet should balance different food groups, including fruits, vegetables, lean protein, whole grains and healthy fats. This balance ensures you get a wide range of essential nutrients.

2. **Variety:** Eating various foods helps you obtain diverse nutrients. Different foods provide different vitamins, minerals and antioxidants, contributing to overall health.

3. **Portion control:** Be mindful of the portion sizes. Eating in appropriate portions can help prevent overeating and maintain a healthy weight.

4. **Whole foods:** Choose whole, minimally processed foods whenever possible. These foods are often more nutrient-dense and contain fewer additives and preservatives.

5. **Fruit and veggies:** Aim to fill half your plate with fruits and vegetables. They are rich in vitamins, minerals, fibre and antioxidants that support good health.

6. **Lean protein:** Include lean protein sources, such as poultry, fish, beans, legumes and tofu. Protein is essential for muscle health.

7. **Whole grains:** Choose whole grains like brown rice, quinoa, whole wheat, and oats, which are higher in fibre and nutrients than refined grains.

8. **Healthy fats:** Incorporate sources of healthy fats, such as avocados, nuts, seeds and olive oil. These fats are essential for brain health and reducing the risk of heart disease.

9. **Limit added sugar:** Reduce consumption of foods and beverages with added sugar. High sugar intake is associated with various health problems, including diabetes, which can lead to weight gain and obesity.

10. **Limit sodium (salt):** Reducing sodium intake can help manage blood pressure and reduce the risk of heart disease.

11. **Hydration:** Stay well hydrated by drinking plenty of water throughout the day. Water has many valuable roles, including assisting digestion, circulation and temperature regulation.

12. **Mindful eating:** Pay attention to your hunger and thirst cues. Eating mindfully can help prevent overeating.

13. **Meal planning:** Plan your meals and snacks to make healthier choices and avoid impulsive, less nutritious options.

14. **Cooking at home:** Preparing meals at home allows you to control the ingredients and cooking methods, making it easier to choose healthier options.

15. **Moderation:** It's okay to enjoy indulgent or less healthy foods occasionally, but everything should be done in moderation.

Now that you understand these 15 key points, I encourage you to review your current eating habits compared to your 'ideal' eating habits and see what you need to improve, add, change and implement before we discuss calories, energy consumption, reading food labels and portion sizes later in this chapter.

ACTIVITY

YOUR CURRENT EATING HABITS

Starting with these questions can help you pinpoint meaningful improvements to help you feel and function your best.

1. What do you consume for breakfast?

2. What percentage of carbohydrates, protein and fats do you consume daily?

3. Do you consume 'bad' fats? If so, what are they and how can you substitute them?

4. Do you eat lunch? If so, is it high in protein?

5. Compare your packaged versus whole foods intake. Which packaged foods could you swap for whole foods?

6. Do you consume fruit and vegetables daily?

7. Do you regularly have any cravings (chocolates, soft drinks, other)?

8. What is your meal frequency? Do you have three main meals and snacks throughout the day?

9. Is your daily structure sedentary?

10. Are you desk-bound?

Remember, it doesn't matter how healthy your food plan is; weight gain will always be a by-product if your calorie intake and portion sizes are too big. All foods contain energy (calories) and extra energy equals weight gain if not used. So, let's examine what calories are, where they come from, the positive impact of calories on human performance and how you can consume calories to suit your lifestyle goals.

Understanding calorie basics

We have all heard about calories, but do you know how many calories you consume daily? I predict 99.9% of you do not, but it is essential to understand your calorie intake when creating your nutritional plan. Why? Calories are energy derived from anything we consume, both food and beverages. They provide fuel for bodily functions, physical activity and general wellbeing. Therefore, to create a sound nutritional plan, it is essential to understand that calories equal energy. Too much energy equals weight gain, whereas too little or a more significant energy expenditure equals weight loss.

So, consider the role of calories as the basic building blocks of energy in your body. The more calories you consume, the more calories you need to burn.

In Chapter 3, we discussed the three main macronutrients, and it is worth understanding that the unit value of a calorie varies depending on whether it is a carbohydrate, protein or fat. Each gram of carbohydrates and protein provides approximately four calories, while each gram of fat provides nine calories.

Do the maths; if you are eating more fat, then you consume more calories. Therefore, by understanding the calorie content of different macronutrients, you can better appreciate their impact on energy intake and make informed choices when constructing a balanced eating plan.

The key is consuming the appropriate calories to maintain a healthy weight, provide adequate energy levels and support overall health. Unfortunately, most of us don't understand the energy balance from the calories we consume through our daily food and beverages, nor the calories expended through physical activity and general bodily functions.

Typically, the average calorie consumption for maintaining a healthy weight in men can vary based on age, weight, height, activity level and metabolism. A general guideline you could work off is 2500–3000 calories per day to maintain weight, assuming a moderate activity level.

The simple equation is when energy intake (calories consumed) equals energy expenditure (calories burned), we maintain weight. If energy intake exceeds expenditure, weight gain occurs. If energy intake falls short, weight loss may occur.

Therefore, you must understand the concept of calorie balance to empower you to make informed choices and decisions to achieve your weight management goal. Your calorie balance refers to the relationship between the number of calories you consume through food and drink and the number of calories your body uses for energy. It's a fundamental concept in managing weight and overall health. When you consume more calories than your body needs, you're in a state of positive calorie balance, which can lead to weight gain over time.

Conversely, when you consume fewer calories than your body needs, you're in a state of negative calorie balance, which can lead to weight loss. Finding the right balance for your body involves understanding your needs based on age, gender, activity level and metabolism. By paying attention to calorie balance and making informed choices about diet and exercise, you can achieve and maintain a healthy weight.

The importance of calorie quality

While the value of calories is essential to understand when designing your nutritional plan, the quality of the calories you consume is equally as important. You may have heard the term empty calories. Regarding nutrition, these refer to the calories in foods and beverages that provide a high-calorie return but offer little to no nutritional value. Typically, these calories are high in added sugar, unhealthy fats and refined carbohydrates, that is, cakes, pastries, cereals, chips and even some smoothies.

The one point I'd like you to remember is that different foods provide essential nutrients, vitamins, minerals and fibre levels. So, eating nutrient-dense foods, such as fruit and vegetables, lean protein, whole grains and 'good' fats, will guarantee that the necessary calories for optimal functioning are consumed consistently. Food variety is an excellent concept to remember when designing your nutritional plan.

Another reason that it is good to understand the value of calories and the type of calories you consume is because it is an essential component of weight management. You need to consider your training goals (weight loss, weight gain, weight maintenance, et cetera) and understand where your calories come from. You should also be aware of the ingredients you are consuming and make sure you are making mindful choices when designing your nutritional platform.

This brings me to the importance of understanding food labels.

Food labels

The power of marketing significantly influences what we consume. When it comes to purchasing healthy food, people are often misled by branding and marketing. We make decisions based on what the food company's marketing team says is good for us rather than making informed decisions based on science.

Therefore, understanding how to read food labels is critical for making informed and healthy food choices. Food labels provide valuable information about a product's nutritional content, including serving size, calories and amounts of various nutrients like fats, carbohydrates and proteins. By understanding the nutritional content and ingredients in what we eat, you can evaluate the food's overall value and make choices aligned with your health goals.

Food labels provide valuable information about packaged foods' nutritional content, ingredients and serving sizes. Although the regulations vary by country, some standard rules and regulations are often followed. Some of the fundamental rules and regulations around food labels include:

1. **Nutritional facts panel:** This includes information on serving size, calories and the amount of various nutrients per serving.

2. **Ingredients list:** Food labels must include an ingredient list that lists all the ingredients in descending order by weight. A general rule I encourage my clients to follow is that the fewer ingredients listed, the better the product.

3. **Allergen labelling:** Food labels must identify any major food allergens, such as peanuts, milk, eggs, fish, soy and wheat.

4. **Health claim:** This might include where the product is made and specific food requirements. If a product claims to be organic or low in fat/sugar, or similar claims, it must meet specific guidelines.

I know there are only four main points. Many people still need to work on reading food labels, so I have created a simple formula for making good food choices and reading food labels easily, allowing you to make informed decisions quickly. I'd suggest eating nothing in a packet in the ideal world, but this is unrealistic today. Still, it is worth considering previous generations and how they consumed foods, particularly seasonal foods and looking at our hunters and gathers that lived on the land. Their body types were lean and muscular, eating protein and seasonal fruits and seeds. Perhaps they even endured periods of fasting, which I will discuss later and definitely NO refined sugar.

Take your time when interpreting the nutritional panel and assess the following:

- **Serving size:** This tells you the recommended portion size for which the nutrient values are provided.

- **Total calories per serving:** Consider this value with your daily calorie needs and weight management goals!

- **Macronutrients:** Identify the amount of carbohydrates, protein and fats.

- **Sugar content:** This is a crucial ingredient for me, as it is associated with various health concerns and lifestyle diseases. Avoid products and ingredients containing corn syrup, sucrose, fructose and other sugar types.

- **Fat content:** Identify the product ratio of 'good' versus 'bad' fats.

- **Sodium:** Be aware of the sodium (salt) content. Packaged foods with a high shelf life contain high levels of sodium/salt.

To simplify reading food labels even further, I encourage you to look at the value of certain ingredients (specifically sugar, saturated fat and sodium) per 100 g or 100 mL and see if the product is of decent quality.

Every food or beverage must be measured per 100 g or 100 mL by law. So, to determine whether the product you are consuming is an 'everyday' food or an 'occasional' food, you need to see if it fits within 'my' guidelines.

The simple formula for reading labels

My simple formula is '5 g–5 g–120 mg per 100 g/mL.'

If the product has 5g or less of sugar (per 100 g or mL), 5g or less of fat (saturated) per 100g or mL and less than 120 mg of sodium (salt) per 100 g or mL, then it is okay. If you compare it to a traffic light, it would be amber, not green or red. It would be a product you can consume every few days, not every day.

If the numbers are significantly higher than 5 g–5 g–120 mg (red zone) or lower than 5 g–5 g–120 mg (green zone), this dictates the frequency of your consumption. Generally, anything in a packet with a long shelf life will be high in sodium.

Nevertheless, remember that food labels are valuable but should be used with other considerations like ingredients, quality and variety. When reading food labels, assessing the marketing claims is equally essential as accurately interpreting the information. This leads me to portion sizes, as regardless of how healthy the calories are, calories and excess calories (energy) equals weight gain, so let's discuss portion sizes.

Portion distortion

Like America, everything in Australia in the 1970s and 1980s had to be significant. Big houses, cars, hair, shoulder pads, pants, steaks and pizzas. Some of you might remember the first mobile phone; it was like a briefcase. Then, as technology progressed, mobiles got smaller and smaller. We kept our mentality around food that the more significant the size the better.

Morgan Spurlock did a fantastic social experiment with his documentary, *Super Size Me*, perfectly reflecting this mindset. After decades of talking, educating and trying to change dietary habits, a large percentage of the Australian population (and the world) is overweight or obese, leading to many lifestyle diseases. The fact is that a large percentage of this is due to portion distortion, overeating of the wrong food groups and the sedentary lifestyle many people lead.

The simple fact is we consume too much energy. You would have seen this when you visit your local café and observe what the public eats. More often than not, an 'Instagrammable' breakfast would include an acai bowl of some description (perhaps with an oversized tablespoon of peanut butter), followed by fresh juice (no fibre) and a coffee, which is around 1000 to 1500 calories for breakfast. Yet their morning exercise probably only burnt off 400 calories at best!

Liquid calories contain an enormous amount of energy, but most people aren't aware of it and wonder why they are not losing weight. The after-exercise meal or beverage is often more significant in calories than the exercise itself. Your portion's size directly impacts your caloric intake, nutrient balance and overall wellbeing.

A well-rounded meal plan should include appropriate portions of carbohydrates, proteins, healthy fats, fruits, vegetables and other essential nutrients. Yet when portion sizes are too large, maintaining this balance becomes challenging, potentially leading to an inadequate intake of certain nutrients.

Below is a snapshot of what two typical structured meal days would look like for me. Consider the combination of all food groups and portion sizes.

My food diary

Day 1

Meal	Food	Protein
Breakfast	150 g oats 30 g protein powder 200 mL whole cream milk (6 g protein)	36 g
Lunch	Salad: 150 g chicken breast (41 g protein), avocado, fetta (10 g protein), olives, cucumber, tomato, rocket, vinaigrette	51 g
Snack	½ cup raw mixed nuts (10 g protein)	10 g
Dinner	150 g salmon fillet (30 g protein) roasted broccolini 1 cup brown rice (4 g protein) ¼ cup slivered almonds (7 g protein)	41 g
Snack	1 cup Greek yoghurt with fresh berries (13 g protein)	13 g
Total Protein		151 g

Day 2

Meal	Food	Protein
Breakfast	Protein smoothie: frozen banana, 2 tbsp nut butter (almond or peanut butter, 4 g protein), 1 tbsp protein powder (30 g protein), 1 cup almond milk (1 g protein), ½ cup blueberries	35 g
Lunch	Prawn salad (6 prawns, 24 g protein), ½ tin mixed beans (16 g protein), avocado, rocket/green leaves, vinaigrette	40 g
Snack	2 boiled eggs (12 g protein)	12 g
Dinner	2 lamb cutlets (36 g protein), 2 small, boiled potatoes. minted peas: 150 g peas (8 g protein), 1 tbsp olive oil, pine nuts (2 g protein), chilli, chopped fresh mint, fetta (2 g protein)	48 g
Snack	1 cup coconut yoghurt/or Greek yoghurt (10 g protein), sliced apple, drizzle raw honey	10 g
Total Protein		145 g

Hit protein numbers and eat consistently

My main focus is constantly hitting my protein number and eating consistently. I also follow a structured training routine of lifting heavy things, including some form of cardio to get my heart rate up.

To control your portion size and help regulate your hunger, consume the protein portion of your meal first and do not overeat. The best start to the day is 150 g of oats with 30 g of protein powder and 200 mL of whole cream milk. This is around 650 calories, with 60 g of carbohydrates, 40 g of protein and 13 g of fats.

Creating a sensible portion size will also help regulate your hunger and fullness cues and control your blood sugar levels, especially regarding carbohydrates. Consuming excessive carbohydrate-rich foods can cause a rapid spike in blood sugar, followed by crashes, which may lead to energy fluctuations and increased hunger. So, controlling portion sizes of carbohydrates can help maintain a more stable blood sugar level. This, in turn, supports a more mindful and intuitive approach to eating.

Statistical trends indicate that our obesity rate will double again over the next 20 years unless we do something about it (*Australian Institute of Health and Welfare* 2024). So, use simple strategies that work for you. For example, if you eat out, you might choose a lunch entree instead of a main meal.

You could also change your eating order. Kickstart your day with protein sources (eggs, yoghurt, smoothie). Eat the protein on your plate first, then your vegetables, and finish with starch foods (potatoes, bread, pasta, rice). Take a leaf out of the French eating habits; their motto is that there is no such thing as 'good' and 'bad' food, just 'sometimes' and 'more often' foods.

Finally, remember to eat slowly and savour your food. It takes 20 minutes for your brain to get signals from your stomach that you are full, so be patient before overeating.

Portion sizes

Understanding portion sizes is crucial for balanced eating and managing overall health. Often, it is easy to underestimate portions, which can lead to unintentionally consuming more than needed. Using everyday objects and hand-based comparisons provides a simple and accessible way to gauge portion sizes without needing scales or measuring cups. This method helps you make mindful choices and avoid overeating.

Here is a guide to standard portion sizes and their hand or object comparisons, making it easier to visualise and control what you eat:

Measurement/food	Comparison
teaspoon	thumb tip or 1 die
tablespoon	thumb or 3 dice
30 g cheese	2 small thumbs or 4 dice
cup	fist or tennis ball
½ cup pasta	small fist or computer mouse
30 g snack food	small handful or small mobile phone
medium fruit/vegetable	fist or tennis ball
80–100 g meat	palm or deck of cards

Using these relatable comparisons, you can manage portions more accurately and support a healthy eating routine.

Portion size, calorie intake and food label awareness are interconnected factors crucial to overall health and wellbeing. Portion control is essential for maintaining a balanced diet and managing weight, helping you regulate calorie intake and achieve proper nutritional balance. You can avoid overeating and make healthier choices by being mindful of portion sizes. Additionally, understanding and interpreting food labels empowers you to make informed dietary decisions, as they provide key details about portion sizes, calories, macronutrients and ingredients.

When designing your healthy nutritional platform, you need to be aware of portion control, the number of calories and food labels. This information will also allow you to make informed choices that promote overall health and wellbeing, not just a short-term energy bump.

Fasting is another popular method for mindful eating and calorie control, so let's explore this.

Fasting

> *Fasting is the greatest remedy; the physician within.*
>
> —**Philippus Paracelsus**

Fasting has gained immense popularity recently as a powerful health and wellness strategy. While it was once a practice rooted in necessity and embraced by various cultures and religions, especially among early hunter-gatherers, today, people choose to fast voluntarily for its potential health benefits.

Many embrace fasting for advantages like weight loss, reduced inflammation, improved insulin sensitivity, calorie control and enhanced metabolic health. They believe it can lower the risk of lifestyle-related diseases and support long-term wellness.

But fasting is not simply skipping a meal now and then—it is a mindful, intentional choice to abstain from eating for a set period. During this time, the body relies on its energy reserves, such as glycogen stored in the liver and fat deposits, to fuel essential functions, encouraging a shift toward more efficient energy use.

There are several types of fasting that you can consider, but before you decide to fast, ask yourself *why* you choose to fast. Is it to control your calorie intake? Is it for health benefits? Is it for spiritual or religious reasons? Is it for mental clarity and focus? Or is it for detoxification and weight loss?

Fasting has been used to improve physical and emotional performance. If it affects your cognitive ability, mood, physical output or stress levels, I suggest another nutritional alternative (there is nothing wrong with a balanced diet). But if it is a simple solution to help you restrict your calorie intake (energy) and drop a few unwanted kilos, then it is worth exploring several types of fasting.

Intermittent fasting types

Intermittent fasting is the most popular method and involves alternating between periods of fasting and eating. This type of fasting often allows for regular eating habits/patterns on non-fasting days or periods. Three distinct kinds of intermittent fasting are structured around the fast versus eating cycle duration.

The intermittent fasting types are:

1. The 16/8 method, where you fast for 16 hours daily and then eat within an eight-hour window. An example of the 16/8 would be skipping breakfast and having your first meal at noon and your last meal at 8 pm. During this fasting period, you can only consume water, tea and black coffee

   By structuring your fasting around 8 pm till 12 noon, you might find it easier to reduce your calorie intake because you are asleep for a substantial portion of the fast. Depending on your 'why' and the reason you are fasting, you need to ensure that when you consume food between 12 noon and 8 pm, you monitor your macronutrient ratio and calorie intake. The same could be said for the 5:2 fasting method.

2. The 5:2 method involves eating normally five days a week and restricting calories to around 500 per day for two days per week. Depending on your preference, these fasting days can be consecutive or non-consecutive.

3. Alternate-day fasting involves fasting every other day, with some variation allowing for limited calorie intake on fasting days. On fasting days, you may either completely abstain from food or limit calorie intake to around 500 calories; regular eating is allowed on non-fasting days.

Prolonged fasting

These three types of fasting are less extreme and more sustainable than prolonged fasting, which typically involves going without food for more than 24 hours.

You may have heard of the water fast; this is an example of prolonged fasting. Both intermittent and prolonged fasting offer distinct health benefits. It is essential that you fast or choose a fasting method that aligns with your health goals, preferences and environmental circumstances. I tried the water fast, lasting three days, but my calorie intake doubled after three days and my macronutrients were out of balance. So, if I were to do any fasting, the 16/8 would probably suit my lifestyle as it is only a means of calorie restriction rather than weight loss.

In Chapter 11, I will focus on 'bio-individuality' and the importance of structuring a health and wellness plan that suits you, as we are all different beings. The same rule applies to fasting and designing your nutritional platform. Fasting has been associated with several potential physical and mental benefits, but does it suit you?

Fasting benefits

The benefits of fasting are the following:

- **Weight loss:** Weight loss is the obvious answer and one of the key drivers of why people choose intermittent fasting. Intermittent fasting restricts calorie intake, leading to a calorie deficit. Through time-restricted fasting, you can reduce your time window for overall calorie intake, facilitating the ability to control your portion sizes.

- **Insulin sensitivity:** Fasting impacts metabolic health markers such as insulin sensitivity, blood sugar control and lipid profiles. One significant benefit of improving your insulin sensitivity is reducing your risk of insulin resistance and Type 2 diabetes.

- **Cellular repair:** Cellular repair is another critical benefit of fasting. During fasting, the body enters a stage described as 'autophagy,' when it breaks down and recycles damaged cells, promoting cellular repair and renewal.

- **Decrease inflammation:** Inflammation reduction is known to be one of the drivers of various health conditions, particularly cardiovascular disease, diabetes and certain cancers. One of the great benefits of fasting is to reduce inflammatory markers in the body, potentially mitigating the risk of these diseases.

- **Brain health:** Fasting increases neuroplasticity, the brain's ability to adapt, recognise and protect against neurodegenerative diseases such as Alzheimer's and Parkinson's.

- **Heart health:** Fasting improves heart markers, reducing cardiovascular disease risk. This, in turn, lowers blood pressure, cholesterol and triglyceride levels.

- **Longevity:** Don't we all want to live longer and be more robust? Fasting might be your answer, as it has been linked to increased lifespan and improved biomarkers, which we know are associated with longevity.

Remember, I am not your fasting expert; I am merely your educator giving you a brief insight into what fasting is. It is crucial to remember that fasting is a dietary practice offering various health benefits, from weight loss to improved blood sugar control and cellular repair. It's only suitable for some and it's crucial to approach fasting cautiously or seek professional help from a qualified expert before you start.

I am not a fasting advocate. Generally speaking, I'm a consistent eater, focusing on eating two grams of protein per kilogram of body weight per day, resistance training four days per week, trying to get seven hours of sleep every night and making sure I drink 150 mL every waking hour. This formula works for me, and more importantly, it is sustainable around my work/family commitments. So, spend time designing your plan and understanding what might work for you. Remember, high performance is personal and about operating at your highest level over an extended period and being consistent.

Let's talk fads

The fitness industry is a multibillion-dollar behemoth, constantly evolving with the latest trends, products and philosophies. Among the most pervasive and profitable sectors are weight loss and nutrition. Unfortunately, this ever-changing landscape often leads to the emergence of fads—trendy diets, workouts and supplements that promise rapid results with minimal effort.

While some of these fads are based on sound science, many are not, leading to cycles of frustration, failure and disappointment for countless individuals. This is probably why I'm employed today. Too many people look for the quick fix or the emotional purchase and then wonder why they don't get the results they want.

The promise of quick fixes is one of the main drivers behind the popularity of fad diets. Whether cutting out entire food groups, drastically reducing calorie intake or embracing the latest superfood, fad diets offer the irresistible allure of rapid weight loss without needing long-term lifestyle changes. Remember what I mentioned earlier: short-term behaviour equals short-term results. When it comes to fad diets, this is particularly true. Some of the most well-known examples include:

1. **The keto craze:** Initially developed as a therapeutic diet for epilepsy, the ketogenic diet has been repurposed as a weight loss tool. By drastically reducing carbohydrates and replacing them with fats, the body is pushed into ketosis, burning fat for fuel. While many experience initial weight loss, the restrictive diet often leads to sustainability issues and potential nutrient deficiencies.

2. **The paleo pursuit:** The paleo diet advocates eating like our hunter-gatherer ancestors, eliminating processed foods, grains and dairy. While its focus on whole foods is commendable, critics argue that it oversimplifies human evolution and neglects that our ancestors' diets varied widely depending on geography and availability.

3. **Detox diets:** Promising to cleanse the body of toxins, detox diets often involve consuming only juices, teas or specific food groups for a set period. Due to their extreme calorie restriction, these diets can lead to rapid weight loss. Still, they also carry risks such as muscle loss, nutrient deficiencies and the potential for eating disorders.

Believe it or not, there is some science behind fads, so it is worth understanding why these diets seem to work temporarily.

Most fad diets share a few common characteristics:

- **Caloric restriction:** Many fad diets result in a caloric deficit, the fundamental principle behind weight loss. Reducing overall calorie intake, whether by cutting carbs, fats or entire meals, often leads to weight loss, at least in the short term.

- **Water weight loss:** Many fad diets cause the body to lose water weight quickly. For example, low-carb diets like keto cause a drop in glycogen stores, which are bound to water in the body. As glycogen is depleted, water is lost, leading to a rapid decrease in weight that is often mistaken for fat loss.

- **Placebo effect:** The psychological impact of starting a new diet or fitness regimen can't be underestimated. Believing that a diet will work can boost motivation, adherence and results—at least temporarily.

Downsides of fad diets

While the immediate results of fad diets can be appealing, they often come with significant downsides. The restrictive nature of these diets can lead to:

- **Nutrient deficiencies:** Cutting out entire food groups or severely limiting calorie intake can deprive the body of essential nutrients, leading to deficiencies affecting everything from energy levels to immune function.

- **Metabolic slowdown:** Prolonged caloric restriction can decrease metabolic rate as the body adapts to what it perceives as starvation. This can make it harder to lose weight and more accessible to gain it back once standard eating patterns are resumed.

- **Mental health impacts:** The cycle of rapid weight loss followed by regain can lead to feelings of failure, low self-esteem and a disordered relationship with food. This yo-yo dieting can have long-lasting psychological effects.

- **Unsustainability:** Most fad diets are not designed for long-term adherence. Once the diet ends, individuals often return to their previous eating habits, leading to weight regain. This cycle can create a sense of hopelessness and frustration, making it harder to achieve lasting health goals.

The fitness industry plays a significant role in perpetuating these fads. Marketing strategies often capitalise on an individual's insecurities and desires for quick results. Celebrities and influencers endorse products and diets, adding to their appeal. In an environment where the next big thing is always around the corner, it's easy to see why people are drawn to these trends despite their potential pitfalls.

Moreover, the industry often neglects to emphasise the importance of bio-individuality, the idea that each person's nutritional needs and responses to exercise are unique. What works for one person may not work for another and this concept is rarely addressed in the one-size-fits-all approach of most fad diets and fitness programs.

Empower yourself with knowledge

So, how can we navigate the noise and make informed choices about weight loss and nutrition? Share *Blokes Inc. Play a Bigger Game* with the masses! Educate yourself and understand what will work for you.

1. **Focus on sustainable habits:** Rather than seeking quick fixes, aim to build sustainable habits that you can maintain long-term. This includes balanced eating, regular physical activity and mindful eating practices. There is nothing wrong with eating the occasional fast-food meal, just don't make it a habit.

2. **Embrace bio-individuality:** Recognise that your body is unique. What works for others might not work for you, and that's okay. Pay attention to how your body responds to different foods and exercises and adjust accordingly.

3. **Seek evidence-based approaches:** When considering a new diet or fitness program, look for those grounded in solid scientific research. Be wary of extreme promises and quick fixes.

4. **Prioritise mental and emotional wellbeing:** Weight loss and nutrition are about the body as well as the mind. Avoid diets and programs that lead to guilt, shame or an unhealthy relationship with food.

5. **Consult professionals:** Registered dietitians, nutritionists and fitness professionals can provide personalised guidance that considers your needs and goals.

Fads in the fitness industry, especially those related to weight loss and nutrition, can be enticing, but I promise you they often do more harm than good in the long run. By understanding the science behind these trends, recognising their risks and focusing on sustainable, evidence-based practices, you can achieve your health goals in a way that supports your overall wellbeing. Remember, the health journey is not a sprint but a marathon that best runs at your own pace, with practices that nourish your body and mind.

Hydration: The vital role of water in health

> *Empty your mind. Be formless. Shapeless. Like water. You put water into a cup; it becomes the cup. You put water into a bottle and it becomes the bottle. You put it in a teapot; it becomes the teapot. Water can flow, or it can crash. Be water, my friend.*
>
> **—Bruce Lee**

I love Bruce Lee's quote about water finding a way. It's so simple yet so accurate. Water can be anything. It has the power, flexibility and tenacity to find a way. I encourage you to do the same.

We take water for granted and the significant role water plays in achieving and maintaining optimal health. Water is not just a simple beverage; it is the essence of life. The human body comprises approximately 60% water and every bodily function relies on an adequate supply of this precious resource. Water is the silent conductor from digestion to circulation, temperature regulation to waste elimination. Without proper hydration, your body will falter and I guarantee most of you are probably walking around dehydrated, day in and day out, yet still functioning. Imagine how you would perform if you were hydrated.

Real-life case: Andrew's dehydration struggles

I recall when my client Andrew reached out and we conducted a three-day nutritional overview. His eating habits were terrible, and his hydration platform was non-existent.

Andrew would wake up at 5 am and have a coffee straight away. If he went to training, he might consume some water, but little water during his session. On his commute to work, he would have another coffee. By mid-morning, he would grab a diet soft drink from the vending machine, thinking he was doing the right thing.

When the 3 pm sugar slump occurred, it was another coffee and a biscuit to energise him before finishing the day with too many beers. It's hard to believe Andrew could function physically and cognitively until it all caught up with him on his commute to Sydney.

More than just water: the importance of electrolyte balance

Andrew was one of the lucky ones. Even in its mild form, dehydration can have far-reaching consequences, impacting physical and mental wellbeing. It is essential when discussing hydration that you don't just think about drinking water. Your body needs a blend of solutions to balance your sodium and potassium with the cells.

I still remember completing my first Comrades Ultra Marathon in South Africa, an 89.9 km race often called the 'ultimate human race.' It is considered the world's largest and most iconic ultra-marathon, steeped in tradition. Not everyone manages to finish, and for some, the extreme challenge proves too much.

The race challenged me physically and mentally and after eight hours and four minutes of running, I reached my goal of becoming a 'Comrade.' After crossing the line, the Bill Rowan medal was placed around my neck and a red rose was handed to me for finishing between seven hours and 30 minutes and nine hours. My vision was a little blurry at this stage and I started to feel faint, but I was now a Comrade, which was my goal. Many people talk about the spirit of the Comrades and to me, this was highlighted as I was leaving the stadium.

A runner had collapsed with 300 metres remaining. He had been running for over 11 hours and his body couldn't keep going. As soon as he fell, two runners following him picked him up and carried him across the line, with one shoulder supporting him. Initially, it was a nice gesture as they were now all Comrades, but for the 33-year-old who collapsed, that would be his last.

Fortunately, it is rare, but it does occur in endurance events. The athlete suffered from hyponatremia, which is when the athlete's sodium (salt) levels drop significantly due to their over-consumption of water. I know it is an extreme example, but unfortunately, this runner thought he was doing the right thing when his lack of education or insight proved his downfall. So, be mindful of your hydration plan.

I have highlighted the worst-case scenario: hydration's critical role in your physical capacity. Firstly, regarding circulation, proper hydration ensures that our blood flows smoothly, carrying essential nutrients and oxygen to cells and removing waste products.

Water also plays a critical role in maintaining body temperature. It allows us to cool down through sweat and conserve heat when it's cold. Water is also a fundamental component of your digestive process, aiding food breakdown and facilitating nutrient absorption. We also know it plays a crucial role in muscle function, as dehydration can lead to muscle cramps and fatigue (sodium and potassium ratio).

Staying adequately hydrated can also help prevent overeating and support weight management as, more often than not, many people eat before they drink. Finally, we all know that a 'hangover' is a feeling of mild dehydration and the effect it has on your mood, potentially leading to feelings of irritability, anxiety and fatigue.

Consume water every waking hour

When in doubt, drink a glass of water. I encourage clients to drink 150 mL per waking hour. More often than not, when you are in an office environment where the temperature is controlled, you rarely proactively drink due for thirst.

Over the many years I have been working with corporate executives, very few have a hydration plan and most operate dehydrated. Typically, they wake up, grab a coffee, commute to work and grab another coffee. Sit in an air-conditioned office all day, have a diet soft drink in the afternoon and then finish the day with an alcoholic beverage or more. Does this sound familiar? Does this sound like Andrew? I don't think he is alone! Reflect on your daily hydration plan. How many glasses of water would you drink between 6 am–6 pm?

Remember, my hourly strategy of 150 mL every waking hour. Regarding optimal hydration, too many variables must be considered (weight, gender, temperature, exercise, environment, sweat rate, and so forth). One of the most apparent physiological measures of your hydration level is the colour of your urine.

Another more accessible indicator is your level of thirst. Typically, if you are thirsty, you are already dehydrated. Hydration is not just about quenching your thirst; it is the foundation of optimal health and wellbeing. Consuming adequate water daily is one of the simplest and most effective ways to support your body's vital physical and mental functions.

By recognising the profound impact of hydration on your life and making it a priority, you take a significant step towards achieving the well-hydrated, vibrant and healthy life you deserve. Now raise a glass to that!

Healthy eating is more than just what you eat

Finally, healthy eating must be addressed when striving for health optimisation. It is the most challenging health dimension to get right, yet it forms the foundation of our wellbeing, impacting our physical health, mental clarity and longevity. Healthy eating is more than just what you eat. It is about the consumption quality, the ratio of your macronutrients, portion sizes, hydration platform and energy expenditure. So, before you design your personalised nutritional blueprint, let's recap the significance of three key elements: variety, macronutrients and fasting.

Variety in our diet is essential because it ensures we receive a broad spectrum of vital nutrients. Remember, protein, carbohydrates and 'good' fats. Balancing these macronutrients in our diet is crucial. Carbohydrates provide energy, proteins are the building blocks for our muscles and tissues and fats are necessary for various bodily functions, particularly brain health. A balanced intake of these macronutrients supports overall health and ensures we have the daily energy and resources to thrive.

Each food group provides unique vitamins, minerals and antioxidants. By diversifying our choices, we can better meet our nutritional needs and make our meals more enjoyable. Healthy eating should be a pleasurable and sustainable habit, not monotonous.

As mentioned earlier, fasting has its place, but I like my food too much, so I focus on portion control and variety as my fundamental foundation. Intermittent fasting and time-restricted eating patterns have gained popularity due to their potential to improve metabolic health and extend lifespan.

In the complex score of life, the importance of healthy eating is the recurring theme that underlines our overall quality of life. The constant refrain influences our physical performance, mental acuity and emotional wellbeing. You can create a harmonious symphony of health and vitality by weaving variety, portion control, macronutrient balance, fasting and hydration into the fabric of your dietary choices.

Remember, the journey towards a healthier, more vibrant life through food is personal. It is not about perfection but progress; whatever your plans are, they must be sustainable. Andrew's plan was more about structure and controlling the controllable.

As you continue to explore the endless possibilities of culinary experiences, remember that healthy eating is an art form we can all master over time, but all artists make mistakes; ask Andrew. In the parlance of many artists, they describe these mistakes as 'happy accidents,' so don't feel guilty if you treat yourself now and then—everything in moderation, except hydration.

Five-step blueprint to improve your nutritional habits

Step 1: Assess your current eating habits

Take a closer look at your current eating patterns.
- Keep a weekly food diary to identify what you eat, when and why you make certain food choices.
- Note unhealthy or overly processed foods, emotional eating triggers and irregular mealtimes.

Step 2: Set clear nutritional goals

- Define specific, realistic nutritional goals that align with your wellbeing objectives. These goals may include consuming more fruits and vegetables, reducing sugar intake or staying hydrated.
- Ensure your goals are measurable and time-bound, such as 'I will eat at least five servings of vegetables daily for the next month.'

Step 3: Plan balanced meals

- Create a well-rounded meal plan that includes a variety of foods from different food groups, such as fruit, vegetables, lean protein, whole grains and healthy fats.
- Pay attention to portion sizes and aim for balanced meals that provide essential nutrients to fuel your body and mind.

Step 4: Make gradual changes

- Instead of drastically overhauling your diet, make small, sustainable changes over time. For example, start by replacing one unhealthy snack with a healthier option.
- Focus on building healthier habits one step at a time, which can be easier to maintain overall.

Step 5: Stay informed and seek support

- Educate yourself about nutrition by reading reputable sources and not believing the marketing food labels.
- Surround yourself with a support system of friends and family who encourage your healthier choices and can help you stay accountable.

Improving your nutritional habits is a continuous journey; patience and forgiveness are essential. Like everything, consistency is the key and there are many food temptations. Nevertheless, following a structured eating plan can make meaningful and sustainable improvements to optimise your overall wellbeing.

What, how, when: the core trio for nutrition and hydration

1. What:

- Define your focus: Identify the specific nutrition, energy and hydration aspects you want to improve. Clarity in your focus areas will guide your actions.
- Nutrition: What nutritional changes do you need? Perhaps increasing your intake of whole foods, balancing macronutrients, or reducing processed foods.
- Energy: What factors affect your energy levels? Consider diet quality, meal timing, and foods that provide sustained energy, such as complex carbohydrates, proteins, and healthy fats.
- Hydration: What are your hydration goals? Determine your daily water needs, considering factors like body size, activity level and climate.

2. How:

- Plan your approach: How you will implement changes in nutrition, boost your energy and maintain hydration? This involves setting up strategies and routines and finding practical solutions.
- Nutrition: How will you improve your diet? Will you meal prep, read labels, incorporate more vegetables, or plan balanced meals with protein, carbs and fats?
- Energy: How will you optimise your energy? Eat regular meals, including protein at breakfast, limit sugar to avoid energy crashes, and balance caffeine intake.
- Hydration: How will you stay hydrated? Will you carry a water bottle, set reminders, infuse water with fruits or herbs for flavour and track your daily intake.

3. When:

- Establish timing and consistency: Specify when you will take nutrition, energy and hydration actions. This will help embed these habits into your daily routine.
- Nutrition: When will you eat? Plan mealtimes that support energy levels throughout the day. Eat breakfast within an hour of waking and space meals and snacks every three to four hours.
- Energy: When will you monitor your energy levels? Remember how you feel after meals, note any energy slumps and adjust your eating patterns.
- Hydration: When will you drink water? Start the day with a glass of water, drink before meals and set specific times, like every hour or after using the restroom, to take a sip.

Take the first step towards lasting wellbeing: create your personalised nutrition and hydration plan

Transform your daily routine by prioritising what, how and when you fuel your body. Building a structured approach to nutrition, energy and hydration does not just support your physical health; it enhances your mental clarity, mood and resilience. Start by choosing nutrient-dense foods that provide lasting energy and balancing your meals to maintain optimal blood sugar levels. Pay attention to timing—well-timed snacks and meals keep your energy steady, especially during busy or active days. Finally, make hydration a habit, as even mild dehydration can sap your focus and energy. Take control of your nutrition today to feel stronger, more alert and ready for anything life throws your way. Start by setting small, achievable goals—then watch how it impacts your day-to-day life.

WRITE DOWN YOUR PLAN HERE:

What:
_____
_____
_____
_____
_____
_____
_____

How:
_____
_____
_____
_____
_____
_____
_____

When:
_____
_____
_____
_____
_____
_____
_____

CHAPTER 5

The art of exercise

As a recovering jock and a qualified exercise physiologist, I am biased when discussing the importance of exercise in your wellness profile. It is one modality that can quickly change your emotional state and has many other physical and cognitive benefits. It is the best form of lifestyle medicine the market can't bottle.

Having worked in the health and fitness industry for well over 20 years, conducting over 30,000 hours as a personal trainer, exercise physiologist, strength and conditioning coach and accountability coach, I have the knowledge and experience to discuss the art of exercise in detail.

In this chapter, I will explore the importance of exercise and delve into its many benefits in pursuing a happier and healthier life. What disheartens me is that most of the population doesn't respect exercise, which is evidenced by the number of people who are overweight or obese, suffer some form of cognitive dysfunction (depression, anxiety) or have inherited one or more chronic lifestyle diseases.

Exercise can minimise, if not eliminate, all of these if they become a constant part of your weekly wellness profile. It is no different from brushing your teeth, showering or making your bed. Exercise must become habitual.

Therefore, in the quest for a longer, healthier and more fulfilling life, few things can rival the transformative power of exercise. Numerous studies show that regular exercise will prevent various diseases, enhance overall wellbeing and positively impact longevity.

A success story: Mark's journey to health

I remember when a client, Mark, walked into my office enquiring about getting a personal trainer. He said, 'I just need a kick start; I know what to do, but I just can't find the time without the financial incentive of paying someone.'

As the words rolled off his tongue, I thought, *wrong answer*! If you want to get fit, lose weight and improve your biometrics, you need to have the intrinsic motivation for it to be sustainable. Mark was adamant that he just needed a kick start, as he had previously been fit, in good health and intrinsically motivated. Over the last decade, Mark's high-stakes career and the associated demands have gradually taken their toll on his wellbeing. I applauded Mark for his honesty and integrity, recognising that he needed to create change, yet from my visual assessment, I knew we had some work to do.

After our initial consultation, I was keen to establish Mark's pain points in an effort for him to become accountable for his own 'personal biometrics' (blood pressure, weight, waist-to-hip ratio and blood profile). Mark knew that to do this properly, his lifestyle drastically needed to shift and I outlined that we could change a few things initially around exercise and nutrition.

Mark's stress profile also needed to be managed. I was very familiar with this type of clientele: highly paid, stressed, underslept, overworked, living off adrenalin with copious amounts of cortisol, yet an attractive bank balance.

For Mark, fast food and alcohol had become a convenient coping mechanism, which exacerbated his weight gain and contributed to his poor sleeping habits. The light bulb moment came when he went for his annual life insurance policy as part of his contract negotiations and the doctor reported that he had gained 15 kilos.

Not only that, but he also had elevated blood pressure, a waist-to-hip ratio outside his parameters, a pale complexion and constant fatigue. My immediate goal was to perform an assessment, including blood work to test and measure his baseline biometrics. This would provide specific feedback to Mark, enabling him to create a starting point for moving forward.

Mark's test results frightened him and placed him at 'high risk.' This typically indicates someone with high blood pressure, a high waist-to-hip ratio, elevated cholesterol and potentially elevated blood glucose. If you don't measure it, you can't manage it, and that is why I put so much emphasis on baseline biometrics when looking for health optimisation.

So, after assessing Mark's blood profile, specific tests raised 'red flags' for me. My immediate plan was to change his environment, reframe his habits and start building behaviours that complemented his long-term goal of living a happy and healthy life, disease-free.

Initially, Mark and I focused on establishing his personalised plan, including achievable fitness goals, a balanced nutritional plan, stress management strategies and supplements to assist his internal operating performance.

Transforming habits for long-term wellness

Mark's commitment to change yielded transformative results quickly. We integrated regular exercise routines into his schedule within the first six-week training block. This included two cardiovascular workouts and two weekly strength training sessions.

I know that once clients start feeling, but more importantly, looking better, their intrinsic motivation and self-care improve tenfold, which was no different for Mark. His attitude shifted considerably. He developed a thirst for knowledge. Everything he did was goal or outcome-orientated. He started eating nutrient-dense foods and replacing his reliance on fast food. He consciously drank less alcohol, which led to improved energy levels and better weight management. He also implemented several stress management techniques, including breath work, visualisation and regular mindfulness breaks during work hours, positively impacting his mental wellbeing.

Mark's newfound commitment to a healthier lifestyle significantly reduced his risk of getting any potential lifestyle diseases associated with prolonged inactivity. Yes, Mark was one of the lucky ones and his journey serves as a testament to the transformative potential of reclaiming health after succumbing to the sedentary lifestyle of a corporate executive.

By simply prioritising fitness, nutrition and stress management, Mark shed over 10 kilos, rekindled his self-esteem and improved his overall wellbeing. A by-product of his weight loss was a significant reduction in his blood pressure, waist-to-hip ratio and his cholesterol (LDL), further highlighting exercise's profound impact on regaining control of one's health and vitality.

The role of exercise in preventing chronic diseases

Mark's story has already highlighted some of the benefits of exercise on one's health. The facts are that regular exercise reduces the risk of chronic diseases such as heart disease, Type 2 diabetes, certain cancers and stroke. I typically classify these as lifestyle diseases, the majority brought on by inactivity and poor nutritional habits.

If you include exercise as part of your weekly routine, it will shield you against chronic disease and positively impact your body's overall health. I am not asking you to exercise daily; I am just encouraging you to add structured exercise into your weekly schedule. Aim for four out of seven days and be consistent.

When doing corporate keynotes or seminars with executives, I often encourage the audience to be, 'Better-Than-Average' and preach the benefits of 'Knowing Your Numbers' (Chapter 6).

Typically, executives respond well to raw data, numbers and spreadsheets. I outline the calendar year (52 weeks) and get them to apply the Better-Than-Average formula to this, aiming for 45 weeks of exercise (structured exercise, which equates to 86%, well above average).

Then, use the same formula weekly. If there are seven days a week, then exercise (structured) four out of seven days (57%). Again, above average. Then do the same for time; if there are 60 minutes in one hour, aim to exercise for 45 minutes. Again, above average, 75%.

Unfortunately, as we age, a large percentage of the population becomes more sedentary; they don't prioritise exercise, mobility or flexibility; they accept that they are getting older and physical deterioration is part of the ageing process.

This attitude frustrates me, yet it is why I get paid well for keeping people alive. I believe in motivating, educating, and holding clients accountable. Lifting heavy things frequently and elevating your heart rate four times weekly with some intensity should be your baseline formula for physical wellbeing. That is before I even mentioned exercise's positive impact on your cognitive health.

Exercise as a cognitive enhancer

Physical activity is effective for managing symptoms of depression and anxiety across numerous populations, including the general population, people with mental illnesses and various other clinical populations. While the benefit of exercise for depression and anxiety is recognised, it is often overlooked in the management of these conditions.

Not only does physical activity trigger the release of endorphins and other mood-boosting neurotransmitters, alleviating stress, anxiety and depression, but it has also been linked to improved memory and focus, playing an essential part in brain hygiene. The cognitive benefits of exercise are not limited to a specific age group. Both children and adults can experience improvements in cognitive function.

Regular exercise promotes the growth of new neurons and increases the production of neurotropic factors. Don't we all want that? Exercise also enhances executive function, which includes higher-order cognitive processes such as attention span, decision-making and problem-solving ability.

Exercise improves attention and concentration by increasing blood flow to the brain, providing it with more oxygen and nutrients necessary for optimal cognitive functioning. Another well-documented benefit is that exercise stimulates the release of neurotransmitters, such as dopamine and norepinephrine, which are the key to improved attention and alertness.

It's also important to note that exercise has a protective effect against cognitive declines and age-related neurodegenerative diseases, such as Alzheimer's disease and dementia.

Exercise promotes neuroplasticity, neurogenesis and the growth of new blood vessels in the brain, which slows the speed of cognitive decline as one ages.

So, before you lace up your shoes and run out the door, let's continue looking at the physical benefits of exercise.

> For me, it's back to 'The Big Three.' Exercise leads to an improved:
> 1. musculoskeletal system
> 2. cardiovascular system
> 3. cognitive function, including memory and focus.

As we age, our bone density decreases (along with everything else). Weight-bearing exercises like walking, jogging, running or resistance/weight training strengthen our bones and can even prevent conditions like osteoporosis by improving bone density and reducing the risk of fractures and bone-related disease.

For some people, regular physical activity can have a huge lifestyle impact as it allows you to maintain independence and improve your functional ability, preserving mobility and balance. So, when designing your personalised exercise blueprint at the end of this chapter, ensure you include cardiovascular/aerobic exercise, resistance/weight training exercises, mobility and VO_2 training into your weekly routine.

Part of the adverse effects of ageing if you don't do any strength or resistance training is the natural decline in muscle mass, known as sarcopenia. By engaging in regular resistance/weight training exercises, you can stimulate muscle growth and help counteract muscle loss, which will, in turn, enhance muscle strength, improve your functional ability and reduce the risk of falls and fractures. And remember, you are always young enough to add muscle if you train correctly and consume a protein-rich diet. The key ingredient is just starting.

Optimising your health through targeted exercise

Regular physical activity has numerous positive effects when optimising your health, including:

- strengthening your heart muscle
- improved circulation
- reduction in blood pressure
- improved blood lipid profile
- weight management
- reduction in inflammation
- enhanced cardiovascular fitness
- stress reduction.

Exercise is not merely a means to achieving a desirable physical appearance or athletic ability; it is a powerful tool for promoting longevity and enhancing overall wellbeing, physically and mentally.

By engaging in regular physical activity and including exercise in your weekly non-negotiables you will enjoy a wide array of benefits, from disease prevention and improved brain hygiene to increased longevity and a higher quality of life. Don't we all want that?

Nevertheless, when considering the specific benefits of exercise, it is essential to understand that they are very subjective to age, gender and health conditions. This is why you need to consider other variables, such as the types, duration and intensity of exercise to suit your 'end goal.' Let's discuss these factors in more detail.

Type of exercise

Creating your personalised exercise blueprint is about tailoring it to your unique needs, goals and desired outcomes—boosting your fitness, dropping kilograms, enhancing athletic performance or preventing diseases. To find the 'best' type of exercise for you, consider your ultimate objectives, your current physical condition and any underlying injuries, illnesses or risks you might have. With that in mind, I recommend integrating a mix of the following modalities into your routine.

Cardiovascular/aerobic exercise

Aerobic exercise, sometimes called Zone 2 training, includes activities that elevate your heart rate and increase your oxygen consumption. These can involve brisk walking (not just on the golf course or while walking the dog), running, cycling or swimming. Aim for an intensity level where you feel slightly uncomfortable—about a six out of 10 on the intensity scale.

While many people may not enjoy it, embracing cardiovascular exercise as a lifelong habit can empower you to take control of your health. It leads to a healthier, happier and more disease-free future. Remember, it's not just about hitting that magical 10,000 steps every day; if weight loss is your goal, it's about how you approach your activities.

Resistance/weight training

I would incorporate resistance training into everyone's blueprint, but very few people lift weights. It doesn't have to involve going to the gym; it could be integrating bodyweight exercises like push-ups, dips, squats, lunges, and bar pulls to begin into your daily routine. Not only does it help build muscular strength, but it will also improve your bone density.

Resistance training is a powerful tool for mitigating the adverse effects of ageing and maintaining physical function, strength and independence as we grow older. By engaging in regular resistance training exercises, you can enjoy the benefits of increased muscle mass, improved functional ability, enhanced cognitive function and an overall better quality of life. Also, your 'activities of daily living' will be a lot easier the stronger you are, not to mention the fact that you are less likely to suffer falls and you will have less chronic pain.

Flexibility

Flexibility is often overlooked but should complement all exercise modalities as it enhances joint mobility and prevents injuries. It might be as simple as incorporating yoga, Pilates or combining structured stretching programs into your daily routine. Just five to ten minutes a day will keep the doctor away.

High-intensity interval training (HIIT)

HIIT has increased in popularity due to a couple of global franchises that have structured their business models around this version of the exercise. This training involves repeated high-intensity bouts followed by varied recovery times. Indeed, it is hard work, and if you have a base level of fitness, your body can manage the load, but I would not recommend this type of training for someone at the start of their fitness journey.

The success or popularity of the franchises is not only due to the type, style or design of the classes but also the social connectivity the brands have created. It is worth noting that many physios have improved their profitability due to the increased popularity of HIIT training.

Understanding the benefits and various types of exercise to include in your personalised blueprint is crucial. But when time is tight, how can you make the most of it? Let's explore the best ways to allocate your exercise time effectively for maximum results.

Duration of exercise

In a society where we are always overcommitting and running from one thing to another, the number one excuse I hear regarding exercise is, 'I don't have enough time.' Yet there are 24 hours a day, 168 hours a week, 52 weeks a year, so time isn't the issue if you prioritise exercise. It is more likely that time management is the real issue. Verbally, most of the population state that they want to look better, feel fitter and function at their optimal capacity, but they aren't willing to sacrifice time to exercise.

When doing corporate keynotes, I often like to reflect on Steve Jobs's last speech before he died:

> *You can employ someone to drive the car for you and make money for you, but you cannot have someone to bear the sickness for you. Material things can be lost and found. But there is one thing that can never be found when it is lost—life.*

He talked about the value of health, love for your family, spouse and friends and the importance of inner happiness and social connectivity. I cannot stress enough the value of creating time to exercise for yourself. Stop looking for excuses and start implementing solutions.

That is why, when working with time-starved executives, I continually challenge them to be 'better than average' and encourage them to run their bodies like a business. In business, some things are 'non-negotiable.' Exercise should be considered just that.

When designing programs for these executives, I encourage them to break down their days, weeks and months and then allocate time for non-negotiables, including exercise, family, social connectivity and down-regulation. I encourage executives to plan their weekly schedule with exercise front of mind. Reframe their thinking to 'but first exercise' rather than 'if I have time.' Exercise needs to be prioritised as you would a meeting, yet the critical component is application and time allocation.

Now, let's explore this concept.

Application versus allocation

Whether you aim to improve cardiovascular fitness, build strength or improve your flexibility, finding the right balance of exercise is essential. When you are goal-oriented, the duration of your workouts directly influences your ability to meet specific goals and objectives, as different fitness goals require varying amounts of time to achieve your result.

If your goal is to improve your cardiovascular fitness, more extended-duration aerobic exercises (running, cycling or swimming) would have to form a large part of your exercise routine. Conversely, if your goal is building muscle, strength training workouts should form the critical foundation of your training program. The same could be said for those who exercise for weight management or abstain from lifestyle disease; consistency is the key.

Also, consider the duration of the exercise based on your experience. If you are commencing your exercise journey, it is crucial to begin with shorter workouts, focusing on building a foundation you can develop before moving forward. Then, as your fitness level improves, you can gradually increase your exercise duration and intensity over time, which is an effective strategy for continual improvement. By understanding your goals, fitness levels, time constraints and preferences, you can tailor your exercise duration to align with your desired outcomes.

If you don't consider 'duration,' then designing your exercise blueprint will affect your ability to achieve your goals. Nevertheless, type and duration are only a few key ingredients that need to be considered when designing your exercise blueprint; intensity is another thing you must consider.

Intensity of exercise

Intensity refers to the effort and energy expenditure level during your chosen activity. There are direct synergies with exercise intensity when it comes to getting results. Your intensity influences your body's physiological and metabolic responses, leading to various adaptations and improvements.

When prescribing a tailored exercise program, I specify the intensity scale starting point related to 'structured' versus 'unstructured' exercise. To simplify this even further, structured training is outcome-orientated or what I describe as purposeful exercise. This would include going to the gym, running, doing a Pilates or yoga class or circuit training. Unstructured exercises include walking the dog, fishing, golf and leisure activities.

Therefore, exercise intensity is critical for a specific goal or result. Whether your goals are weight management, cardiovascular fitness or strength, finding the appropriate level of intensity is vital. It is also imperative to understand the relationship between exercise intensity and its impact on your body, as this will enable you to tailor your workouts to optimise results, enhance your performance and reap the benefits of higher-intensity training.

More often than not, most of the population don't exercise at all, let alone at the appropriate exercise intensity and then they wonder why they are not getting the results they are after. If you exercise at the same intensity for the same duration, your body will get used to the physiological stress and plateau under the same load. This is why the critical variable you need to alter is time and intensity to create stress, which will challenge your body to create an adaptation.

Several factors determine exercise intensity, including heart rate, exertion, breathing rate and even the amount of weight or resistance used. In 1970, Dr. Gunnar Borg developed the Borg Rating of Perceived Exertion (RPE) scale, as a subjective measure to gauge an individual's perceived exertion during physical activity. The Borg scale ranges from six to 20 and each numeral corresponds to a description of exertion (see below).

6—7:
Exceptionally light. No exertion at all.

8—10:
Very light, barely noticeable exercise.

11—12:
Fairly light. Light effort, comfortable.

13—14:
Somewhat challenging. It is a noticeable effort but still sustainable.

15—16:
Hard. It is an arduous effort but still manageable.

17—18:
Arduous. Arduous effort, uncomfortable.

19—20:
Maximal exertion. The maximal effort, unsustainable.

As an exercise physiologist, I understand the Borg scale and during my university days, we used it frequently during testing protocols. When I used it for the general population, the Borg scale was a little hard to quantify, so I simplified it and used a 0–10 scale. (0 equals sitting on the couch and 10/10 was exhausted, gasping for breath). This method is more subjective and relatable and allows individuals to self-regulate.

When considering your intensity scale, you should consider three primary levels to ensure you have the right balance of intensity to suit your fitness levels, goals and overall health.

1. **Low-intensity:** Low-intensity exercise refers to elementary activities and things you can do for an extended period. This might include walking, stretching or a casual bike ride. While low-intensity exercise is sustainable for beginners or those recovering from injury, it wouldn't provide significant health benefits if you hope to improve your cardiovascular health or strength. On my 0–10 intensity scale, for example, the low intensity would be anywhere between 0–3.

2. **Moderate-intensity:** Moderate-intensity exercise increases your heart and breathing rates, making you feel like you are doing something. This might include jogging, circuit training, a boxing circuit or purposeful cycling. It is a more 'structured' exercise with a meaningful outcome. During this phase, you get physiological benefits, such as calorie burning, improved cardiovascular response and strength gains. Typically, when referring to my scale (0–10 intensity), you would be between 4–7/10 during this intensity phase.

3. **High-intensity:** High-intensity training is when you push your body to its maximum capacity. This should contribute around 10% of your weekly training load, described as VO_2 training. It's that feeling when you sprint that last 150 metres of your run. Your breath rate and execution level are high and require significant effort and energy. Typically, many of you would be

familiar with HIIT; this is high-intensity training that challenges your cardiovascular system. For many, particularly beginners, this phase is too hard, unsustainable and can cause injuries. Your heart rate is high, so you can't sustain a conversation. You are right at your threshold on the intensity scale, 8–9/10.

When designing your exercise blueprint, it is critical to approach intensity and duration gradually and systematically. For many of us, being uncomfortable is tough and maintaining accountability is more arduous, which is why the personal training industry has thrived.

A good personal trainer will design a tailored program to suit your needs, set the intensity levels and modify your program to ensure you achieve your desired outcomes/results.

Zone 2 (moderate) and VO_2 max (high-intensity interval) training must be a critical blend to optimise your health and physical fitness.

Zone 2 training is characterised by moderate intensity, which enhances your aerobic capacity, promotes fat metabolism and builds a solid endurance base. When you exercise in Zone 2, you can sustain your output for extended periods, supporting your overall cardiovascular health and energy efficiency.

VO_2 max training involves short bursts of high-intensity effort, pushing the body to its maximum oxygen uptake. This training improves anaerobic capacity, increases metabolic rate and boosts cardiovascular efficiency, but it is extremely uncomfortable and why most people don't do it.

By incorporating moderate and high-intensity workouts, you can achieve a balanced fitness regime that maximises endurance, strength, and metabolic health. This will improve performance and increase the likelihood of long-term wellness.

Therefore, consider what you are training for. Suppose you want to burn calories, control weight or manage weight. In that case, higher-intensity exercise will lead to greater calorie consumption post-workout as your resting heart rate will be higher for longer. This is referred to as your post-exercise oxygen consumption (EPOC). This is why HIIT and

VO_2 training is valuable for weight loss. If dropping a few kilos is your desired result, include HIIT training in your exercise blueprint if your body can cope with the demand.

High intensity for happiness

Engaging in 'structured' moderate-intensity exercise improves cardiovascular fitness and reduces chronic disease risk. While another recently well-documented benefit of intensity training is its influence on psychological wellbeing. Studies have shown that engaging in high-intensity exercise/activities triggers the release of endorphins, which are feel-good hormones (Basso et al., 2017).

There is enough evidence to suggest that there is a direct correlation with intensity, mood, your level of stress, your mental clarity and your ability to cope. Reflect on that feeling when you achieve something you didn't think was possible. The sense of achievement, accomplishment and improved confidence leads to a positive mindset.

Having worked in the health and fitness industry and studied human behaviour for over 20 years, I have witnessed numerous clients who neglected their health dedicating all their time to their profession, which includes Mark. Some were lucky enough to act and implement a strategy before it was too late.

At the same time, unfortunately, others paid the fatal price of using and abusing their health as a commodity. Then, it came time to retire; they were financially rich but physically and emotionally bankrupt. This is why I preach to all my clients to run their bodies like a business and constantly perform a regular health audit, test, measure and understand their biometrics so a proactive plan can be implemented if there is an abnormality.

Enough evidence supports the benefits of exercise, which extend well beyond physical fitness and encompass mental, emotional, and cognitive aspects of health. Regular exercise can and will enhance cardiovascular health, strengthen muscles and bones, maintain weight, and reduce the risk of chronic disease. Exercise is not just a means to maintain physical fitness but also a crucial ingredient for a long, happy and healthy life.

Finding the 'f for fun' in fitness

Like any human behaviour, it will not be sustainable if we don't like something. So, the key is to find the 'f for fun' in fitness because you won't stay consistent if you don't like it. So, let's look at your options around various exercise modalities. Understand that all modalities have benefits, but your chosen modality needs to align with your exercise goal/s and desired outcome/s.

The crucial ingredient is the fun component. It may take some trial and error until you feel you have the framework that suits you to build on.

Exercise modalities

Here is a list of some of the different exercises that would fit under each of the exercise modalities.

1. Cardiovascular (aerobic) exercise includes:

- running
- walking
- cycling
- swimming
- rowing
- HIIT classes/sessions
- boxing.

2. Strength training exercise includes:

- weight training
- bodyweight exercises
- resistance bands
- kettlebells.

3. Flexibility exercise includes:

- yoga
- Pilates
- stretching
- tai chi.

4. Balance and stability includes:

- balance exercises
- BOSU balance trainer exercises
- Swiss ball/fitball exercises.

5. Functional training exercises that mimic movements used in your chosen sport or daily activities.

6. Group fitness classes includes:

- spin
- aerobics
- boxing
- circuits
- other structured classes.

The key is to align your preferences with your goal/s and remain consistent.

So, now is your time to create your individualised exercise blueprint. Enhance your longevity and enjoy exercise's countless benefits for your health and wellbeing.

Tips to help you design your blueprint

Designing a personalised fitness blueprint is essential for achieving your health and wellness goals. Whether you aim to build muscle, lose weight, boost overall fitness, enhance sleep quality, develop athletic skills, lower health risks, manage pain or improve mobility, a clear, structured plan can make all the difference. The guide below provides key tips to help you shape an effective blueprint for success.

1. Start by identifying your goals. Your main goals may be to:
   - increase muscle
   - decrease weight
   - improve fitness
   - improve sleep
   - develop athletic skills
   - reduce risk profile
   - reduce pain
   - improve mobility

2. Think about your time allocation.

3. Consider which modalities you will use.

4. Identify any potential roadblocks.

5. Plan your weekly training sessions, allocating four out of seven days to scheduled exercise.

6. Review your frequency.

Five-step blueprint for improving exercise habits

Step 1: Set clear, personalised goals

Start by defining your exercise goals precisely. Are you aiming to lose weight, build muscle, improve cardiovascular health or feel more energised? Then, tailor your goals to your current fitness level and personal interests.

Use the SMART criteria (Specific, Measurable, Achievable, Relevant, Time-bound) to set goals that motivate and guide you. For example, 'I will walk for 30 minutes, five days a week, for the next month' is a clear and achievable goal.

Step 2: Find activities you enjoy (finding the 'f for fun')

The best exercise routine is one that you look forward to. Explore different forms of physical activity to discover what you enjoy most—weightlifting, cycling, yoga, hiking or playing a sport. Enjoyment is essential to consistency, so prioritise activities that bring you joy and fit your lifestyle. Mix it up to keep things exciting and to work different muscle groups, which can help prevent boredom and overuse injuries.

Step 3: Schedule your workouts

Treat exercise like any other necessary appointment. Block out specific times in your calendar for workouts and stick to them as you would with meetings or social engagements.

Consistency is built through routine, so find a time of day that works best for you, whether it's early morning, during lunch breaks or in the evening.

Starting with shorter, more manageable sessions can help establish the habit without feeling overwhelmed.

Step 4: Track your progress and celebrate wins

Track your workouts and progress to stay motivated and accountable. Use a fitness app, journal or simple checklist to log your activities, duration and any changes in how you feel.

Set small milestones and celebrate your achievements, no matter how minor they seem. Recognising progress reinforces positive behaviour and keeps you motivated to continue.

Step 5: Prioritise recovery and listen to your body

Optimal wellbeing is not just about exercise but also about recovering and caring for your body. Incorporate rest days into your routine to allow your muscles to repair and grow.

Pay attention to signals from your body, such as fatigue, soreness or lack of motivation, which might indicate a need for rest or a change in routine. Focus on adequate sleep, proper nutrition, hydration and stretching to support your wellbeing and exercise habits.

Following this five-step blueprint, you can develop sustainable exercise habits that improve your physical fitness and overall wellbeing. These habits will make you feel stronger, more energised and more resilient in your daily life.

Remember, consistency is the critical ingredient in improving exercise habits. Start small and gradually increase the intensity and frequency of your workouts. Once you start gaining, your body will require another stress response, so continually change your blueprint.

Celebrate your progress and be flexible in adapting your plan to align with your wellbeing goals.

What, how, when: the core trio for exercise habits

1. What:

- Define your exercise goals: Start by clearly identifying what you want to achieve with your exercise routine. Having a clear focus will guide your actions and keep you motivated.
- Exercise habits: What specific habits do you want to build? Examples include exercising three times a week, increasing your daily steps or incorporating strength training.
- Wellbeing optimisation: What aspects of your wellbeing are you targeting? Consider goals like reducing stress, boosting energy levels, improving sleep or enhancing mental clarity.

2. How:

- Plan your approach: Determine how you will achieve your exercise and wellbeing goals. This involves setting up actionable steps, strategies and routines that fit your lifestyle.
- Exercise habits: How will you implement these habits? Create a workout plan, choose activities you enjoy, set realistic and progressive targets and use tools like fitness apps or classes to guide you.
- Wellbeing optimisation: How will you ensure your exercise supports your overall wellbeing? Incorporate a balanced mix of cardio, strength, flexibility and relaxation exercises like yoga or stretching. Ensure your approach includes aspects of recovery, like adequate rest and nutrition.

3. When:

- Establish timing and consistency: Specify when you will engage in exercise and activities that support your wellbeing. Consistency is vital, so establish a routine that integrates seamlessly into your daily life.

- Exercise habits: When will you exercise? Choose days and times that work best for you—such as early mornings, lunch breaks or evenings. Consider setting a consistent schedule, like exercising every Monday, Wednesday and Friday, to build a reliable habit.
- Wellbeing optimisation: When will you check in on your wellbeing? Schedule moments for reflection, like weekly reviews of how you feel physically and mentally. Adjust your exercise routine based on your energy levels, sleep quality and mood.

Take the first step towards lasting wellbeing: create your personalised exercise plan

Achieve lasting wellbeing by focusing on what, how and when you exercise. A balanced, transparent plan that aligns with your lifestyle is critical to consistency and optimal results. Start by choosing exercises that match your goals and energy levels, paying attention to how each workout fits into your day—whether it is a brisk morning walk or an evening gym session. A structured approach will keep you consistent and ensures each workout strengthens your health and happiness. Commit to prioritising your wellbeing today; take that first step and see how a thoughtfully planned exercise routine can uplift your entire life.

WRITE DOWN YOUR PLAN HERE:

What:

_____
_____
_____
_____
_____
_____
_____

How:

_____
_____
_____
_____
_____
_____
_____

When:

_____
_____
_____
_____
_____
_____
_____

CHAPTER 6

Know your numbers

When asked what surprised him most about humanity, the Dalai Lama answered, 'Man! Because he sacrifices his health to make money. Then he sacrifices money to recuperate his health.'

If you look at the latest data, it is alarming that 66.9% of Australians are classified as overweight or obese and 12% are categorised as severely obese, which is associated with a body mass index (BMI) over 35 (*Australian Institute of Health and Welfare* 2024). Many people may argue that the statistics are inaccurate, but unfortunately, the facts are the facts.

The impact of excess weight on health

Enough evidence and scientific data indicate that excess weight correlates directly with all-cause mortality. Extra weight has a direct correlation with increased blood pressure/hypertension, Type 2 diabetes, osteoarthritis, sleep apnoea, many cancers, depression and general body pain, restricting one's activities of daily living.

I have often asked clients, 'How is your blood pressure?' The typical response is, 'My doctor says it's okay.' Well, what is okay? What is your blood pressure? The facts are that most of the population would know their weight in kilos and/or their bank balance, but they do not know any of their vital health biometrics.

When assessing my clients, I take specific measurements and then educate them on the cause and effect of such biometrics, resting blood pressure being one of them and body weight another. I want to see their blood pressure when their heart rate is elevated or when their heart is stressed. What is their diastolic blood pressure response?

As I mentioned in earlier chapters, to optimise one's health, running one's body like a business is imperative. To do this, numbers/data are critical to analyse because if you don't test and measure it, you cannot manage it.

This is why personal health accountability and regular monitoring are essential components of longevity. Numbers need to be contextualised and understood. Many of you need to understand your numbers, so in this chapter, I will address the critical biometrics I would like you to understand, test and track as part of your health audit.

The importance of proactive health monitoring

Understanding and knowing your numbers means you can create a proactive management plan and possibly prevent health issues. Regularly tracking personal biometrics, such as heart rate, blood pressure, glucose levels, waist-to-hip ratio, weight and sleep patterns, can detect any early signs of abnormalities, giving you time to create a preventative plan of action.

Awareness of your biometrics will mean you can make informed decisions based on your 'at risk' biometric data. If required, you can actively modify your lifestyle choices, such as diet, exercise, sleep and stress management, enhancing your overall wellbeing.

Over the years working in the executive health space, I have found that personalised health data empowers people to collaborate more effectively with health professionals. This ensures that tailored interventions and treatments accurately align with improving one's health profile.

Personal health monitoring bridges the gap between reactive healthcare and proactive wellness. Reactive healthcare involves responding to health issues and diagnosing and treating illnesses after they manifest, typically the roles of doctors. My goal throughout this book is to prevent this.

This approach often results in higher costs and more intensive medical interventions. If I can educate and motivate you to 'take ownership', know your numbers and regularly test and measure your biometrics, you can minimise your risk. This proactive approach would include implementing regular exercise, creating a balanced nutritional plan, establishing a sleep hygiene strategy, implementing stress management techniques and participating in routine health audits.

I do not doubt that prioritising a proactive wellness plan will enhance your quality of life, reduce significant healthcare expenses and achieve better long-term health outcomes. Don't we all want that?

Throughout this chapter, I will educate you on the importance of regular testing and encourage you to 'know your numbers' to keep you accountable, but more importantly, physically and mentally healthier.

Regardless of how fit you think you are or your level of apprehension towards testing, it is essential that we collect some baseline fitness biometrics. Don't worry about the numbers; focus on your goal (improved functionality, decreased stress, pain reduction, weight loss, improved fitness, muscle gain, etc). Early detection can save lives, so make your biometrics your business.

Case study: Mark's health transformation

In Chapter 5, I discussed Mark as an example of someone consumed by the corporate merry-go-round to the detriment of his health. Mark's subsequent health biometrics would have certainly increased his risk profile and could have easily led to many types of chronic illness had he not proactively changed his environment/lifestyle. This is why it is essential to regularly test your biometrics, as it allows you to minimise your reactive health risks.

You can then implement a strategy to reduce ongoing health issues by identifying potential hazards. The only way to do this actively is by placing your risk profile through your raw data, hence my affiliation with biometric testing. This is why I constantly encourage you to run your body like a business, as the same principles of management, strategy and continuous improvement are required. Just as a business relies on accurate financial statements to understand its profit and loss, your biometric testing results gain insights into your health biometrics.

Biometrics, such as blood pressure, cholesterol, glucose and other vital signs, resemble a business's financial indicators. Without understanding your health biometrics, it's challenging to implement specific changes to improve your performance and overall wellbeing.

Knowing your profit and loss allows you to identify areas needing attention and create strategies for growth and efficiency in a company. Similarly, regular biometric testing provides valuable data about your body's condition, enabling you to make informed diet, exercise, sleep and stress management decisions.

Mark knew he was overweight; he could see that and noticed his suits and pants no longer fit. His shirts were tighter, his face puffier and his complexion reflected someone who was continually fatigued. However, he didn't know his lifestyle's significant impact on his biometrics (elevated blood pressure, cholesterol, glucose). Typically, I evaluate and measure every six weeks and then suggest yearly, more extensive health audits.

After Mark's initial health audit identified his lifestyle risk factors, we created a specific six-week training block, considering his work and travel commitments. After Mark completed each six-week training block, we would re-test his basic biometrics, resting heart rate, weight, blood pressure and waist-to-hip ratio, and analyse his results. Based on that information, we would establish specific goals for the next six weeks around his exercise frequency, daily nutritional requirements (including any supplements), and ability to down-regulate.

To Mark's credit, he continued to show progress every six weeks showing positive results, which were enough to maintain his intrinsic motivation, and his pants were finally looser.

I remember reviewing Mark's annual health audit after we received his biomarkers from his GP. Not only had he shed the excess weight he desperately wanted to, but he had also revitalised his physical fitness and, more importantly, experienced a significant boost in his self-esteem.

His results reflected his improved lifestyle choices, and his blood profile was now all 'within range,' after starting in the 'red zone' for BMI, waist measurements, weight and blood pressure. He also had a few blood markers that were 'within range' but on the higher side (cholesterol, calcium score, and blood glucose).

When analysing Mark's results, I remember he was shocked that he was considered 'at risk.' We discussed the impact of his lifestyle on his health profile and the dangers that could occur if a specific plan was not implemented.

Mark's results typified those of a corporate executive: high BMI, high blood pressure, and high cholesterol, which I refer to as the 'unhealthy triad.' His diastolic high blood pressure was greater than 90 (ideal is 80), his waist-to-hip ratio was above 0.90, and his bad cholesterol was 4.2 mmol/L (optimal is less than 2.6 mmol/L).

Although outside of the guidelines and alarming for Mark, these markers are more often than not a direct result of poor lifestyle choices and are 100% reversible. If they are not addressed, they can potentially lead to increasing your risk of chronic disease (heart disease, stroke, Type 2 diabetes, to name a few).

Mark's results showed that his current lifestyle was significantly having an impact on his health. If I had not tested Mark's biometrics, I would not have had the raw data that allows me to give constructive feedback on the direct effect of Mark's lifestyle choices on his biometrics.

Mark's results are not uncommon. They represent the 'unhealthy triad': increased weight gain, increased waist measurement, increased blood pressure, and, often, increased blood lipid profile. These biometric indicators are typically related to a poor lifestyle. Without the initial testing phase, it would be challenging to validate a poor lifestyle's impact on one's health other than the visual and physical (lethargy) impact.

Getting personal health data can intrinsically motivate lifestyle changes by providing a clear, tangible insight into one's health status. When individuals see their biometric measurements—such as elevated cholesterol levels, high blood pressure, high body fat percentage and high glucose levels—they better understand how their daily habits impact their wellbeing. This personalised information is a powerful wake-up call. It fosters a sense of accountability and empowers individuals to take control of their health.

With accurate, personalised data, people are more likely to adopt healthier behaviours, such as regular exercise, improved nutritional habits and effective stress management techniques, as they can quantify the benefits these changes bring to their biometric markers. This continuous feedback loop of data and improvement motivates people to maintain a healthy lifestyle, highlighting the importance of knowing their numbers.

Getting clients to complete their blood profiling is vital to their health audit. Similar to assessing your business's profit and loss statement, blood profiling provides a comprehensive insight into various aspects of your health that are not always apparent through external symptoms or general wellness checks. By analysing a range of biomarkers present in the blood, blood profiling can offer a detailed picture of your physiological and metabolic processes.

Why blood profiling is essential for long-term wellness

Although I have the utmost respect for doctors, it is worth noting that when they are conducting blood tests, typically, they are treating sick patients and looking for any markers outside of the 'normal' reference range that may have an impact on one's 'disease state' or the patient's current state of health, rather than treating a deconditioned executive who is just looking to optimise their health, as in Mark's case.

Most doctors reviewing Mark's blood profile would say his results are all within range or borderline. But for me, this isn't proactive enough. My goal is to minimise any future risk of any potential disease in the future.

From my visual examination of Mark, I saw that he was overwhelmed. From this observation I could also assume he would have higher than recommended blood pressure, which could align with his increased waist-to-hip ratio. Mark's poor lifestyle choices over the last 12–18 months had a significant impact on his health (weight gain, decreased cardiovascular fitness), but the only way I could accurately assess this was by testing his blood.

Here are key reasons why blood profiling is essential:

1. **Detection of hidden conditions:** Blood tests can reveal underlying health issues such as diabetes, thyroid disorders, anaemia, infections and high cholesterol levels, often before symptoms manifest. Early detection allows for timely intervention and management.

2. **Nutritional status:** Blood profiling can identify deficiencies in essential vitamins and minerals, such as Vitamin D, iron and Vitamin B. Understanding these deficiencies helps tailor nutritional plans and supplementation to address specific needs.

3. **Hormonal balance:** Hormones regulate various bodily functions, including metabolism, mood and energy levels. Blood tests can assess hormonal levels and identify health and wellbeing imbalances.

4. **Inflammation and immune function:** Chronic inflammation is linked to numerous health conditions, including heart disease, arthritis and autoimmune disorders. Blood profiling can measure inflammation markers, helping identify and manage these risks.

5. **Liver and kidney function:** Blood tests provide essential data on liver and kidney health, vital for detoxification and waste elimination. Monitoring these functions can prevent and manage diseases related to these organs. Typically, corporate executives put their livers and kidneys under duress due to poor nutritional habits and alcohol consumption.

6. **Cardiovascular health:** Another factor correlating with poor nutritional habits and weight gain is increased cholesterol and lipid levels. Therefore, it is essential to test these markers and make informed decisions about diet, exercise and medication to reduce the risk of heart disease and the impact on one's cardiovascular health.

7. **Personalised health optimisation:** Understanding one's unique biological markers allows individuals to create highly personalised health plans, which is imperative. This targeted approach ensures that any interventions you implement, such as dietary changes, exercise regimens, and lifestyle adjustments, are tailored to your needs.

Once you have received and assessed your results, you can implement an action plan to improve any markers that may be elevated, borderline or on the higher side of the range.

Typically, if clients are within range or on the higher side of 'normal,' it doesn't give them the sense of urgency that most of the population needs. My approach is 'shock now, save later'! Implementing a preventative plan by modifying one's lifestyle choices is easier before any potential lifestyle disease is prevalent.

Therefore, step one is conducting your health audit through physical assessment and blood profiling. Step two is assessing the results and understanding any risk markers. Step three is crucial—implementing changes to optimise your physical and cognitive potential.

Personal health audit

Blood pressure

Blood pressure measures the force exerted on your artery walls as your heart pumps blood through your body. It is recorded with two numbers:

- **Systolic pressure (the top number):** This represents the pressure in your arteries when your heart beats and pumps blood. Stimulants like caffeine, nicotine or energy drinks, which increase heart rate, can fluctuate this number.

- **Diastolic pressure (the bottom number):** This shows the pressure in your arteries when your heart rests between beats. Because it reflects the resting pressure, I focus on the diastolic number, as it offers a clearer picture of the baseline strain on your arteries and is less affected by temporary changes in heart rate.

Ideal blood pressure range

An ideal blood pressure reading is around 120/80 mm Hg (systolic/diastolic). A diastolic reading above 90 mm Hg can indicate high blood pressure or hypertension, which may need lifestyle adjustments or medical intervention to reduce health risks.

Waist/hip (W/H) ratio

Your waist-to-hip ratio is your waist measurement in centimetres divided by your hip measurement in centimetres. The higher your ratio, typically, the greater the chance of certain disease or diabetes.

Ideal waist-to-hip ratio range

0.80–0.95

Body mass index (BMI)

BMI is calculated by dividing weight in kilograms by height in square meters. A high BMI can mean a person is overweight or obese. It would be best to consider the individual's waist measurement, as sometimes shorter, more muscular men have a higher BMI but aren't overweight. These individuals are more often than not described as mesomorphs.

BMI ranges

> 18.5–24.9 is considered healthy.
> 25–29.9 is considered overweight.
> 30+ is considered obese.

Complete blood count

The complete blood count test examines the different cells in your blood, including red and white blood cells and platelets. It looks for abnormalities in your blood that help diagnose various illnesses, infections and diseases (anaemia, heart disease, iron deficiency, autoimmune disorder or, worse, cancer).

Basic metabolic panel

The basic metabolic panel test helps check the body's fluid balance and electrolytes by examining kidney function. A basic test would consider calcium, carbon dioxide, chloride, creatine, potassium, sodium and urea nitrogen. The calcium score is the main number I focus on as it reflects calcium deposits in the heart. When calcium is present, the higher the score, the higher the risk of heart disease.

Metabolic panel ranges

A calcium score of 0 means there is no evidence of heart disease.

> 1–10 is minimal evidence of heart disease.
> 11–100 is mild evidence of heart disease.
> 101–400 is for moderate evidence of heart disease.

Lipid panel

In laypeople's terms, this test looks at the amount of fat in your blood, measured as the amount of cholesterol and triglycerides.

Lipid panel ranges

Your numbers should be:

> Total cholesterol under 200 mg/dl
> LDL under 100 mg/dl
> HDL over 60 mg/dl and
> Triglycerides under 150 mg/dl

C-reactive protein

The C-reactive protein test checks for inflammation in your body, such as rheumatoid arthritis, lupus or Crohn's disease.

C-reactive protein ranges

> 0.3 mg/dl is the average level seen in most healthy adults.
> 0.3 to 1.0 mg/dl is normal or slightly elevated.

Testosterone

I love this test when we discuss men's health as it shows much more than the sex hormone. Ideally, it is tested first thing in the morning at its highest. Studies have shown that decreased levels have been linked to obesity, fatigue, depression and sarcopenia (loss of muscle mass from ageing), not to mention a reduced sex drive and erectile dysfunction. Typically, it is age-related, which is another reason I like it tested as we get older.

Testosterone ranges (nanograms per decilitre)

Age 20–24: 409–558 ng/dL
Age 25–29: 413–575 ng/dL
Age 30–34: 359–498 ng/dL
Age 35–40: 352–478 ng/dL

It is important to note that, unfortunately, a man's testosterone level peaks at age 20 when the average is 679 ng/dl.

Weight

Regular monitoring of body weight can help track changes over time, providing insight into the effectiveness of dietary habits, exercise routines and lifestyle choices. Maintaining a healthy body weight is crucial for reducing the risk of numerous health conditions, including heart disease, diabetes and hypertension. It also plays a significant role in maintaining proper metabolic function and hormonal balance.

Moreover, understanding and managing your body weight can improve energy levels, mobility and mental wellbeing. By monitoring this essential metric, you can make informed decisions and necessary adjustments to support your long-term health and wellness goals.

Why testing

My passion for motivating men comes from working in the health industry for over 20 years and noticing that men are less proactive about acting for their health than women. So, for those men reading this book, I encourage you to become a 'MACS' (Men Always Consult Someone). The first step might be simply speaking to one of your close friends about a health issue that concerns you. Speak openly and honestly with your doctor and take your first step to personal health accountability.

It is imperative to understand the impact that your lifestyle choices might be having on not only your physical health but also your mental health. Like anything, the first time is the most daunting. Still, once you have initiated and completed your first health audit, the aim is to compare your tests year on year, making sure your lifestyle isn't negatively affecting your health, unlike Mark's.

I cannot stress the importance of regular biometric testing to maintain optimal health or, at the very least, minimise the impact of any potential lifestyle diseases. This is why I put so much value on 'knowing your numbers.' By monitoring your biometric measurements, such as your weight, BMI, waist-to-hip ratio, and blood profiling, you can take proactive steps toward reducing risks.

I cannot recommend biometric testing enough. The associated results should then form the framework of your exercise and nutrition blueprints.

Five-step blueprint for improving your biometrics

Step 1: Assess your current baseline

Begin by understanding your current health status through a comprehensive biometrics assessment. This may include critical metrics such as weight, body mass index, body fat percentage, blood pressure, cholesterol levels, blood glucose and fitness tests. You can do this through a health check-up with your doctor, wearable devices or apps tracking these metrics. Knowing your baseline provides a clear starting point and helps identify areas that need improvement.

Step 2: Set specific, measurable goals

Set specific and measurable health goals tailored to your needs based on your baseline data. For example, you might aim to reduce your body fat percentage, lower your blood pressure or improve your aerobic fitness. Use the SMART criteria (Specific, Measurable, Achievable, Relevant, Time-bound) to create clear and attainable goals. For instance, 'Reduce my body fat percentage by 5% in six months by exercising four times a week and adjusting my diet.'

Step 3: Develop a personalised action plan

Create a personalised action plan that addresses key areas such as nutrition, exercise, sleep and stress management.

- Nutrition: Focus on a balanced diet of whole foods, vegetables, lean proteins, healthy fats and adequate hydration. Consider consulting a nutritionist to tailor your diet to your specific needs.
- Exercise: Incorporate cardiovascular, strength and flexibility training to improve overall fitness and biometrics.
- Sleep: Aim for seven to nine hours of quality sleep each night, as poor sleep can negatively impact your biometrics.
- Stress management: Practice stress-reducing techniques like meditation, deep breathing or engaging in hobbies.

Step 4: Monitor your progress regularly

Track your progress consistently by measuring your biometrics at regular intervals. Use wearable technology, apps or scheduled check-ups to monitor key health indicators. Regular monitoring allows you to see improvements, identify trends and adjust your plan if necessary. Keeping a health journal or using apps to log your data can help maintain motivation and accountability.

Step 5: Adjust and optimise your approach

Health improvement is an ongoing process, so be prepared to adjust your plan based on your progress and changes in your life. Don't hesitate to modify your approach if specific strategies aren't yielding results. Seek professional guidance when needed, such as consulting with a fitness coach, dietitian or healthcare provider to refine your strategy and optimise your efforts. Continually revisit your goals, celebrate your successes and set new targets to keep progressing toward an optimal health profile.

By following this five-step blueprint, you'll create a structured, actionable plan that improves your biometrics and enhances your overall health and wellbeing, empowering you to live a healthier, happier life.

What, how, when: the core trio for personal biometrics

1. **What:**

2. Identify key biometrics and health metrics: Start by defining the specific ones you want to focus on. This clarity will guide your actions and help you set meaningful goals.

3. Biometrics: What are the key metrics you need to monitor? Consider body fat percentage, weight, blood pressure, cholesterol, blood glucose levels, resting heart rate or VO_2 max.

4. Health profile: What overall health aspects do you want to improve? This might include improving cardiovascular health, reducing body fat, enhancing physical fitness or managing stress.

2. How:

- Develop your action plan: Determine how you will improve your biometrics and health profile. This involves setting up specific actions, routines and strategies tailored to your goals.

- Biometrics: How will you measure and improve these metrics? Use a combination of regular health check-ups, wearable tech (like fitness trackers) and apps that track progress. Develop a balanced approach with diet, exercise, sleep and stress management tailored to your goals.

- Health profile: How will you create a holistic plan for overall health? Integrate personalised nutrition, exercise routines (including strength, cardio and flexibility), consistent sleep schedules and stress reduction techniques like mindfulness or yoga. Adjust your plan based on feedback from your biometrics.

3. When:

- Set a consistent schedule for monitoring and action: Specify when you will act and monitor your progress. Consistency is crucial for making lasting improvements in your health profile.

- Biometrics: When will you measure your biometrics? Set regular intervals, such as weekly or monthly, to track changes and assess progress. For example, check your weight and body fat percentage weekly and schedule blood tests quarterly or twice yearly.

- Health profile: When will you implement your action plan? Establish a consistent daily or weekly routine, including exercise, meal planning, and mindfulness practices. For example, commit to exercising every Monday, Wednesday and Friday at 7 am or set aside Sunday afternoons for meal prep.

Take the first step towards lasting wellbeing: create your personalised biometrics and health profile

Take control of your health journey by focusing on the what, how and when of your personal biometrics and health profile. By building a focused, actionable plan, you will keep track of your progress and gain insights that help you make informed, data-driven choices. Think of each metric—sleep quality, blood pressure or fitness levels—as a valuable tool for understanding and enhancing your wellbeing. This approach empowers you to improve continuously, fine-tune your health routine and create lasting, positive changes. Start today with a plan that truly supports your long-term vitality.

WRITE DOWN YOUR PLAN HERE:

What:
_____
_____
_____
_____
_____
_____
_____

How:
_____
_____
_____
_____
_____
_____
_____

When:
_____
_____
_____
_____
_____
_____
_____

CHAPTER 7

Sleep is not a tradable commodity

The importance of sleep for health optimisation

Some people love it, some crave it, some can't function without it, yet plenty of people abuse it. We all desperately need sleep to live a happy and healthy life. Sleep is an essential ingredient if you aspire to health optimisation.

Sleep should not be considered a luxury; it is a vital component of a healthy lifestyle that should be prioritised along with nutrition and exercise. Many people overlook sleep's importance and adopt a casual 'I'll sleep when I'm dead' attitude. In today's fast-paced, always-connected world, it is common for individuals to sacrifice sleep for work, social obligations or entertainment. Yet, research consistently demonstrates that sleep is vital in promoting optimal health and wellbeing.

So, if you are someone who disrespects sleep, then at some stage, your body will disrespect you. During this chapter, I will highlight that sleep is an indispensable aspect of human existence, impacting every facet of our lives, from physical wellbeing to mental health and overall quality of life.

Case study: John and the Corporate Struggle

I remember a great client of mine, John, whom I trained for around five years. He contacted me after I did a presentation at his workplace. I vividly remember the presentation I used that day: 'Know Your Numbers, For Health Optimisation.' This presentation is structured to inspire, educate, and motivate executives by shedding light on the importance of understanding and monitoring critical health indicators.

During the presentation, I delved into compelling population statistics. I emphasised the urgency of proactive health measures by providing a comprehensive overview of health issues resulting from poor lifestyle choices. My goal was to educate executives about the potential risks their lifestyles may pose and then inspire them to take concrete actions toward healthier behaviours.

By fostering an awareness of individual health metrics, executives can make informed decisions and cultivate sustainable habits that enhance their wellbeing and professional effectiveness. Something in the presentation hit a chord with John, who approached me for details after I finished.

I called John soon after and I remember a tone of vulnerability in his voice. At the time of the conversation, John was only 41 years old and had plenty of time to correct his bad behavioural habits before they became an issue. I reinforced his bravery in reaching out and suggested a 'lifestyle' consultation to establish some background information that might paint the picture of why he was noticing a decline in performance.

I needed to understand his daily behaviours to identify his habits. I needed to know whether he was exercising and, if so, the intensity, frequency and specificity of the exercise. I also needed to access his daily/weekly alcohol intake, his sleep hygiene, and any other stressors (work or family) that might impact his operating system.

At John's first assessment with me, I'd describe him as your typical corporate exec, entangled in the demanding web of a high-stress job, excessive work hours, and poor sleep habits. His thirst for professional recognition meant he would frequently burn the candle at both ends, working long hours to meet deadlines and show the firm he had leadership capabilities.

This behaviour is not ideal, but the physical and physiological symptoms are reversible if addressed early. When it becomes prolonged, the stress and side effects grow more serious. Over time, the cumulative impact of late nights, poor sleep habits, lack of exercise, excessive alcohol or medication and fast food can turn short-term issues into chronic conditions, putting your long-term health at risk.

This is precisely the situation John found himself in. His health was starting to suffer, initially marked by weight gain, fatigue, and a noticeable decline in cognitive performance. John became aware of this because he noticed a sense of lethargy. He observed that the frequent tasks he used to do now took 20% longer. John felt he didn't have the mental clarity he once had, which he described as brain fog.

Caffeine was the only way he could kick-start his cognitive function. He knew exercising and eating correctly could reduce his weight, but he lacked the motivation to start. Previously, John had signed up to his local gym, but like 90% of the population, he didn't use it; his membership was merely a donation to the gym owner.

John's journey: a wake-up call for lifestyle change

Nevertheless, John knew something needed to change, and the first step was identifying the problem/s and then working out a plan of action. This is no different from a work situation; if there is a problem, there must be a plan to resolve it.

With work-related tasks, executives excel, identify problems, and then implement solution-based outcomes. Yet, when the problem is personal, they neglect the number one asset. This is why I encourage you to run your body like a business. The accountability solution-orientated approach is transferable. Remember, if we can measure it, we can manage it.

In John's case, the problem was he was one-dimensional—100% work focused—but he was determined to reclaim his vitality.

After our initial consultation, I saw that John's signs and symptoms were 100% reflective of his poor health behaviours, which were 100% reflective of his employment. Initially, I wasn't concerned about the extra kilos around his waist or the frozen pizza John was heating up after work every night.

I was concerned about John's lack of sleep—less than six hours per night. I was concerned about the stress and the potential impact this could have on John's health and mortality. I was also worried about

John's demanding job, often leading to late nights at the office. These combined stressors meant that he struggled to unwind and disconnect from work and the only effective way he felt he could disconnect and relax was to self-medicate with alcohol.

Sleep became a luxury for John, with only a few hours allocated each night. The persistent sleep deprivation took a toll on his physical health, which led to weight gain. I was adamant that this behaviour and John's lack of sleep were causing the decline in his cognitive abilities and his overwhelming sense of lethargy.

After identifying what we believed had the most significant impact on his current lifestyle, we planned to embark on a transformative journey to identify his stressors, improve his sleep hygiene and establish healthier habits.

John was no different from many other corporate executives who don't value sleep. The statistics show that if you let your ego shape your attitude, you will become another number and never reach your lifestyle potential, personal and professional. Fortunately, this 'I'll sleep when I'm dead' attitude did not excite John, so we implemented a four-step process to reframe his current lifestyle to positively impact his behaviour.

Embracing technology: wearables and sleep tracking

Step one was to reframe or retrain John's brain to realise the importance of sleep and the impact that a lack of sleep has. Along with some education, John's thirst for change increased tenfold and he became focused on consciously changing his sleep hygiene.

Over the years, I have found that an effective way to motivate executives is to provide data directly related to their physiological functioning/output. When it comes to sleep, I love the use of wearables.

Step two was to get John to embrace technology and use a wearable. The advantage of this is that wearable devices have advanced sleep-tracking capabilities, which offer users valuable insights into their nightly sleeping patterns, including sleep duration, quality and disturbances. By leveraging this data, I have found that clients can better understand their sleep behaviours and identify improvement areas. For John, this data—his data—with real-time monitoring and feedback empowered him to make informed lifestyle adjustments, which in turn fostered better sleep hygiene.

For many of my corporate executive clients struggling with stress management or sleep apnoea, I have found integrating technology into their daily routine gives them intrinsic motivation but, more importantly, validation of the importance of sleep. Using wearables in the quest for improved sleep aligns with our modern, fast-paced lives but also serves as a proactive and personalised approach to achieving a more restful and rejuvenating night's sleep. Once the wearable has gained enough data to support and validate poor sleeping habits, the critical phase is integration, leading me to step three.

Step three is the important phase from validation to implementation. Typically, I like to gain two weeks' worth of data, which gives enough feedback about my client's sleep behavioural patterns. This allows me to formulate a structured sleeping routine based on my client's work and environmental factors. To improve one's sleep hygiene, we must create a sustainable solution. Sleep requires a conscious effort and level of commitment to create change.

Assessing John's sleep data showed a consistent pattern of poor, broken sleep routines. John's sleeping patterns were slightly better on the weekends, but deep rapid eye movement (REM) sleep quality still needed improvement. The weekends showed improved bed rest but not necessarily improved non-rapid eye movement (NREM) or REM sleep cycles, and my focus was to get John to sleep through more 'complete' sleep cycles.

From data to action: implementing effective sleep hygiene

After highlighting this data, John made a conscious effort to change his sleeping habits, which was particularly important for me as I have little control over this behaviour once my clients are home. I constantly preach it but can't enforce it; the intention is one thing, yet implementation, action and commitment to change are critical ingredients that must be intrinsic for lasting change.

It wasn't just a matter of going to bed at the same time every night to improve John's sleeping habits. Many other variables needed to be considered as well, including artificial light, nutrition, hormonal imbalance, gut issues, exposure to screen time and, when ready for bed, the room environment, temperature, light and noise.

We established boundaries around screen time, lighting, food and time to improve John's sleep routine. Initially, I set John a realistic yet potentially challenging goal of seven hours of sleep per night. I wasn't interested in the total hours in bed; I was more concerned about the number of sleep cycles John had.

Therefore, John's new routine involved:

1. Creating a calming bedtime ritual.

2. Disconnecting from electronic devices 90 minutes before sleep.

3. Creating a dark and comfortable sleep environment of around 16–18 degrees Celsius.

I got John to fill in a sleep diary for the next two weeks to track his progress and articulate his feelings. This way, we could accurately cross-reference his sleep quality and physiological functioning. Having worked with many executives suffering similar symptoms to John, I find the first two to four weeks particularly important as this is typically when clients are intrinsically motivated to create change.

John quickly identified patterns and potential disruptors by diligently recording daily sleep patterns, including bedtime, wake time, caffeine intake and screen usage before sleep. Once we assessed this data, it was just a matter of changing John's pre-bedtime routine to cultivate a better sleep hygiene environment.

Self-awareness is instrumental in recognising habits that may adversely affect sleep quality. I love using sleep diaries, as they are a tangible record you can share with healthcare professionals, facilitating a more accurate assessment of your sleep issues.

Tracking emotions, stress levels, daily activities, and sleep patterns in the diary allows for a holistic understanding of the factors influencing sleep. The data is even more compelling if done in correlation with a wearable device.

Step four was the final stage, acknowledging the new habit formation based on a sound sleep hygiene routine. For John, this phase highlighted his level of commitment. We had enough data, and his consistency validated his feedback. The impact of his improved sleep hygiene techniques and his dedication to improving his sleeping habits was nothing short of transformative.

In just a few weeks, he experienced a remarkable improvement in his physical and cognitive wellbeing. Not only did John immediately notice he was feeling better with reduced fatigue, but he was also making better, more informed decisions around his wellbeing, nutrition and exercise routine. Finally, John was becoming multidimensional.

When John initially contacted me and completed his lifestyle consultation, he agreed to commit to an eight-week training block. The initial focus was to identify which lifestyle behaviours had the most significant impact on his health, and then the plan was to retrain and reframe his behavioural habits. We agreed that sleep, specifically a lack of sleep, significantly impacted his current health status.

Over the next eight weeks, John consciously tried to improve his sleep hygiene. Within three weeks, his metabolism regulated and he became more energised throughout the day. John's cognitive performance witnessed a ten-fold improvement; his focus sharpened and his decision-making became more precise, supported by the data retrieved from his wearable.

The improvement in John's wellbeing was not limited to physical and cognitive aspects alone. His stress levels significantly decreased, and he found a newfound balance in his life. The ripple effect of adequate sleep extended beyond night hours, positively influencing his mood, interpersonal relationships and overall quality of life.

John's initial eight-week training block with me lasted beyond five years when he joined my accountability program. Weekly training, scheduling, optimising nutrition and staying physically and emotionally fit became habitual.

By recognising the importance of rest and making intentional changes, John not only reversed the adverse effects of sleep deprivation but also unlocked a level of wellbeing that transcended his initial expectations. This is another example that validates the transformative potential of prioritising sleep toward optimal health and vitality.

Sleep is critical for maintaining physical health and improving cognitive functioning, emotional wellbeing and overall vitality.

Now that you have read John's story and how a lack of sleep affected his physical and emotional wellbeing, reflect and review your sleeping habits. How is your cognitive health?

Look at a few ways that you could improve your sleep hygiene. You will thank me for it in the long run.

ACTIVITY

1. Circle a number from 1 to 10 (extreme value) on how you rate sleep.

   1   2   3   4   5   6   7   8   9   10

2. Now, circle the average hours you sleep a night, Monday through Thursday (ideally, it should be the same across seven days).

   4   5   6   7   8   9   10+

3. Now, circle the average hours you sleep a night, Friday–Sunday.

   4   5   6   7   8   9   10+

4. Now, write down the total number of hours you sleep in a week.

The art of sleep

Adequate sleep contributes to physical and mental wellbeing, cognitive function and productivity, so it is essential to respect the benefits sleep has on your body. This is why it is important to understand the stages of sleep cycles and then look at ways to improve your sleep hygiene. I always preach to my clients that knowledge and understanding are only one aspect, but like exercise and nutrition, implementation is the key and when it comes to sleep, it should be no different.

The benefits of a good night's sleep

As John's story identified, sleep has many physical benefits but let's look at the impact from birth until death. Think of infants and the number of hours they sleep. Infants have higher sleep requirements as sleep is critical for growth, development, and physiological needs, from the formation of new neurons to physical growth, the release of growth hormones and the maturation and functioning of the immune system. Sleep is critical for optimal development from infants onwards.

Sleep is a fundamental biological necessity for all humans and creatures. Like everything I have discussed in previous chapters, sleep cycles have natural variability and flexibility (bio-individuality). Some people can go 24 hours without sleep and in the right circumstances without lasting harm.

If a person is deprived of sleep for an extended period, several mental and physical problems may begin to develop. Sleep plays an essential role as we age, from growth and development in the early stages to therapeutic and healing benefits. Therefore, we must respect, continually strengthen and aim to maintain a robust immune system.

Unfortunately, many of the lifestyle diseases the population faces today have a direct relationship with inadequate sleep, as sleep deprivation has been shown to lead to high blood pressure and even the increased likelihood of developing cardiovascular diseases, such as stroke or heart disease and more recent studies looking at it as a significant risk factor for dementia (Torres et al 2007).

A good night's sleep can balance our hormones, particularly cortisol (the stress hormone) and promote the release of our happy hormone, endorphin. We also know that when it comes to aesthetics, your sleep duration and quality of sleep are intricately linked to weight management, reinforcing its relationship with hormone regulation. If you sleep poorly, you more often than not have increased hunger and more significant cravings associated with weight gain and the increased risk of obesity. Sound familiar?

More importantly, quality sleep is linked to optimal mental and emotional health. The more time your head is on the pillow, the greater your cognitive health (attention, concentration, memory). During sleep, the immune system performs a host of vital regenerative functions necessary for the optimal functioning of a healthy mind and body.

Consider your brain as a computer. Sleeping at night is like pressing Control-Alt-Delete, clearing and preparing the brain for the next day. It demands downtime to do this properly; your internal body clock is undergoing an IOS upgrade. You can't function optimally if you don't allow your mind to switch off.

We all know that feeling when you haven't slept enough. You might be a little more irritable, you might have more mood swings, be less tolerant of others around you and could potentially have more significant anxiety. When we lack sleep, our emotional control is jeopardised and many of you who have had kids would understand how a lack of sleep clearly expresses heightened emotions with irritability. I know when I was juggling the art of becoming a new dad and had three kids under four, sleep was a luxury, as such my moods changed dramatically and my work output dropped significantly.

Effects of sleep deprivation

It is no wonder that sleep deprivation has been used as a form of torture treatment for decades. There are many reported cases around torture treatment and sleep deprivation, yet for ethical reasons, when we look at science and research, there is a limit to how far you can push human subjects. Some researchers have used animals, and the studies have shown physiological failure and, in extreme circumstances, death. This indicates that the entire body requires adequate physiological and psychological rest.

Reflect on a time when you have suffered a form of sleep deprivation due to work, travel, family and/or social commitments and the cognitive and physical effects it had on you the following day. Imagine the compound effect sleep deprivation would have on you over time—the unpleasant feelings of fatigue, irritability and difficulty concentrating. Then, under more extreme circumstances, problems with reading and speaking, poor judgment, lower body temperature and a considerable increase in appetite will manifest.

If sleep deprivation continues over an extended period, then the corresponding worsening side-effects occur, which include disorientation, visual misperceptions, apathy, severe lethargy and social withdrawal. There is no way you would even consider going for a run, doing weights or cooking a healthy meal under extreme fatigue.

Therefore, optimal sleep is associated with a longer and healthier life, so I encourage you to look at changing your 'sleep when I'm dead' attitude and respect that sleep is a fundamental pillar of wellness, critical for maintaining not only physical health, but also improved cognitive functioning, emotional wellbeing and overall vitality.

In Chapter 5, I discussed planning your exercise blueprint around your work commitments and sleep is no different; a sleeping schedule should be followed and maintained as much as possible, Monday through to Sunday. You have to form complementary habits that last. When you design your optimal sleep routine, you should create a consistent plan over seven days, not just Monday to Thursday, when your week follows a work routine. I like the old saying, 'early to bed, early to rise.' Bed by 9 pm and up at 5 am is a solid eight hours.

How many hours do you get per night?

What is your sleep routine?

I constantly preach it; implementation, action and commitment are the three critical ingredients needed to create change.

Lifestyle factors affecting sleep

Before I discuss the sleep cycle stages and how each stage impacts how we look, feel and function, let's consider a few lifestyle factors that may influence your sleep quality.

Unsurprisingly, regular physical activity promotes better sleep by helping regulate the sleep-wake cycle and reducing stress. The old saying 'you are what you eat' is also true, as diet plays a critical role in the quality of sleep you get. Heavy meals, such as high-carbohydrate foods (starchy products), can interfere with falling and staying asleep and spike your insulin level. Certain beverages can also impact your sleep. The obvious ones would be caffeine and alcohol, but sugary drinks can also affect your sleep quality.

Additionally, exposure to screens and bright lights before bed can suppress melatonin production, making it harder to fall asleep. So, to improve your sleep hygiene, aim for natural light in the morning, which increases your morning cortisol levels and then again towards the end of the day, as natural light helps increase your melatonin.

Unfortunately, the office environment doesn't provide such options. Many corporate executives live under bright artificial lights in a stressful climate, causing their cortisol levels to remain high throughout the day and suppressing any potential melatonin production. The best way to combat this is to get outside early in the morning and expose your eyes to the sun.

By maintaining a consistent sleep schedule and controlling your exercise routine, nutrition, bedroom environment and work environment, your body's internal clock will self-regulate, making it easier to fall asleep. If your sleep hygiene needs to improve, assess your daily routine from morning to evening. Consider how you could make minor improvements to impact your sleep quality positively. Consider your current sleep environment and the impact this might have on your sleep cycles. Identify the negative environmental habits that need to change and then work on a strategy that allows you to implement positive actions that will lead to positive behavioural change.

Stages of sleep cycles

To optimise your sleeping habits and improve your sleep hygiene, let's explore and understand the stages of sleep cycles. This will give you a greater understanding of the complexity of sleep and why sleep is not solely determined by the time your head is on the pillow but by the number and duration of the sleep cycles you experience every night.

Typically, a sleep cycle consists of two main phases repeated throughout the night, each with unique characteristics and functions. The first phase is non-rapid eye movement (NREM) sleep, which accounts for approximately 75–80% of the entire sleep cycle and is broken down into three distinct stages: N1 (light sleep), N2 (main stage of NREM) and N3 (deep sleep).

N1 is the transition between wakefulness and sleep. You can probably associate your behaviours during this phase when you are just starting to nod off; your brain activity is slowing down, yet you can wake up quickly. This is a brief stage, lasting only a few minutes.

N2 is the main stage during your NREM phase, accounting for 50% of your total sleep time. This is when your brain activity slows even further. During N2, your body enters a deeper state of relaxation, your body temperature drops, your heart rate drops and your breathing becomes regular.

N3, also called 'deep sleep,' is the most essential stage of the NREM cycle. This stage usually occurs during the first half of the night and its duration decreases as the night progresses. During this deep sleep phase, your brain waves, commonly called your delta waves, which are responsible for tissue repair, growth and hormone regulation, slow down. It is challenging to wake you when you are in the N3 phase. This deep sleep phase is critical for physical restoration, immune function and wellbeing.

Once you have completed the NREM phase of your sleep cycle, you then move into the REM stage, which occurs approximately 90 minutes after falling asleep and, as it states, is characterised by rapid eye movements, increased brain activity and vivid dreaming. This stage of your sleep cycle is critical for various cognitive functions and emotional regulation. It is an exciting stage as your brain becomes highly active, like in your wakeful state. However, your body is in a state of temporary paralysis, called 'REM atonia.' Throughout the night, your sleep cycles repeat themselves, each lasting 90–120 minutes, and as you progress, your REM sleep increases while your NREM sleep decreases.

I often talk to my clients about the importance of sleep, which I highlighted with John's story earlier in this chapter. Although I am not a sleep expert, I understand the physiological benefits of each stage of the sleep cycle and neither the NREM nor REM sleep cycle have a higher level of importance. Both cycles play a crucial role in your body's optimal level of functioning. NREM sleep promotes physical restoration, while REM sleep supports cognitive and emotional wellbeing. This is also why I encourage my clients to use wearables, particularly at the beginning, so they can look at their data, assess their sleep cycles and validate the duration of NREM sleep versus REM sleep.

The balance and quality of the overall sleep cycle are critical factors in promoting restful sleep and reaping the benefits of the 'complete' sleep cycle. Completing multiple sleep cycles throughout the night is the key, as waking up in the middle of a sleep cycle, especially during deep sleep, can lead to that feeling of grogginess.

Ideally, the average person goes through four to six complete sleep cycles a night and you know my theory about being 'better than average,' so let's work out roughly how many cycles you are going through. For example, each cycle lasts approximately 90–120 minutes, so the average is 90 minutes. Ideally, I'd love you to sleep seven and a half to nine hours per night (bed by 9 pm and up at 5 am), meaning you would go through five to six complete sleep cycles.

Many clients struggle with sleep, particularly when I encourage them to become 'better than average.' Developing a routine is the quickest and easiest way to improve sleep. My initial advice is to try and establish a structure around sleep. Start by going to bed at the same time and then getting up at the same time, Monday through Sunday. Remember, the bedroom is for sleeping or copulating, preferably both, consistently.

Nevertheless, like many other physiological variables, there are always outliers and some people (very few) don't need six sleep cycles to function adequately and feel rested. Generally speaking, your body's performance response will allow you to gauge the 'ideal' number of sleep cycles you need. That is fine if you think you can work physically and cognitively well off five to six hours a night. Yet, plenty of evidence suggests less than six hours significantly impacts how you look, feel and function physically and emotionally. I respect the demands of work and family life, but sustained periods of sleep deprivation will catch up on you, so please be mindful of not just the time in bed but also the number of sleep cycles you have daily. Either way, the compound effect will determine your optimal performance outcome.

Now that you have a greater understanding of the benefits of quality sleep and the importance and complexity of your sleep cycles, you need to embrace the value of sleep as an essential pillar of a healthy lifestyle.

Developing a personalised sleep schedule

Developing a personalised sleep schedule and integrating relaxation techniques before bedtime can significantly improve sleep quality and wellbeing. Develop a calming bedtime routine that signals your body that it's time to wind down. This can include activities like reading a book, practising gentle stretching or doing relaxation exercises.

Remember that developing a personalised sleep schedule and incorporating relaxation techniques is a journey. Finding what works best for you may take time, so be patient and consistent. Making sleep and relaxation a priority can improve sleep quality and overall health and wellbeing.

Five-step blueprint for improving sleep

Step 1: Establish a consistent sleep schedule

The foundation of good sleep is consistency. Set a regular bedtime and wake-up time, even on weekends, to regulate your body's internal clock. This consistency helps improve the quality of your sleep over time. Aim for seven to nine hours of sleep each night, depending on your needs. Gradually adjust your schedule in 15-minute increments to reach your ideal sleep and wake times.

Step 2: Create a relaxing bedtime routine

Develop a calming pre-sleep routine to signal your body that it's time to wind down. This could include reading, taking a warm bath, meditating or practising gentle stretches. Avoid stimulating activities, screens and bright lights at least an hour before bedtime, as these can interfere with your body's natural production of melatonin, the hormone that regulates sleep.

Step 3: Optimise your sleep environment

Your sleep environment plays a crucial role in the quality of your rest. Keep your bedroom calm, dark and quiet to ensure it is conducive to sleep. Invest in a comfortable mattress and pillows suited to your sleep preferences. Use blackout curtains, earplugs or white noise machines to minimise disruptions. Keep electronics out of the bedroom and reserve your bed for sleep and relaxation.

Step 4: Manage diet and physical activity

What you eat and how active you are can significantly affect your sleep. Avoid large meals, caffeine and alcohol close to bedtime, as these can disrupt your sleep cycle. Engage in regular physical activity during the day, as it promotes better sleep, but try to finish vigorous exercise at least a few hours before bedtime to avoid overstimulation. Light, relaxing activities like walking or yoga close to bedtime can help promote relaxation.

Step 5: Address stress and mental health

Stress and anxiety are common culprits of poor sleep. To clear your mind before bed, practice stress management techniques such as mindfulness, meditation, deep breathing or journalling. If worries keep you awake, try writing down your thoughts to release them before sleep. If sleep problems persist, consider seeking professional advice or therapy to address underlying stress, anxiety or other mental health concerns.

Following this five-step blueprint can create a solid foundation for improving your sleep quality, leading to better overall health, increased energy and enhanced wellbeing.

Like every chapter, consistency and patience are the keys to implementing change, and altering your sleeping habits/environment is no different.

What, how, when: the core trio for sleep

1. What:

- Define your sleep goals: Start by identifying the specific aspects of your sleep that you want to improve. Understanding your sleep needs and challenges will help you tailor your approach.

- Sleep goals: What do you want to achieve? This could include getting seven to nine hours of quality sleep, falling asleep faster, reducing nighttime awakenings or feeling refreshed.

2. How:

- Develop your sleep strategy: Determine how you will improve your sleep quality. This involves setting up routines, making environmental adjustments and adopting healthy sleep practices.

- Sleep environment: How will you optimise your sleep space? Make your bedroom conducive to rest by keeping it cool, dark and quiet. Use blackout curtains and white noise machines and ensure your mattress and pillows are comfortable.

- Bedtime routine: How will you prepare for sleep? Develop a calming pre-sleep routine that includes reading, a warm bath or practising relaxation techniques such as deep breathing or meditation. Avoid screens and bright lights at least an hour before bedtime to reduce blue light exposure.

3. When:

- Set consistent sleep and wake times: Specify when you go to bed and wake up to establish a regular sleep schedule. Consistency helps regulate your body's internal clock, making it easier to fall asleep and wake up naturally.

- Sleep schedule: When will you go to bed and wake up? Aim to go to bed and wake up simultaneously every day, even on weekends. For example, set a bedtime of 10 pm and a wake-up time of 6 am to ensure eight hours of sleep.

- Pre-sleep routine: When will you start winding down? Begin your bedtime routine about 30—60 minutes before your designated sleep time to signal your body that it's time to relax and prepare for rest.

Take the first step towards lasting wellbeing: create your personalised sleep plan

Transform your nights and energise your days by focusing on the what, how and when of your sleep. With a structured, actionable plan, you will uncover the habits and routines that can make quality sleep a consistent part of your life. This approach helps you prioritise rest, ensuring you wake up refreshed and with the energy you need to tackle your day and improve your overall wellbeing. Embrace the power of better sleep—start today with steps that truly impact your health and daily performance.

WRITE DOWN YOUR PLAN HERE:

What:
_____
_____
_____
_____
_____
_____

How:
_____
_____
_____
_____
_____
_____

When:
_____
_____
_____
_____
_____
_____

CHAPTER 8

That dirty word 'stress'

Stress emerges as a powerful motivator and a potential adversary in the intricate tapestry of men's health. The key is to harness the good and eliminate the bad. I love the saying 'pressure is a privilege.' When we refer to stress, we must also understand that some stress is necessary.

Moderate stress can drive productivity and resilience, helping you to perform at your best under pressure. In the corporate sector, I have seen the profound negative impact chronic stress can have on your health—from cardiovascular disease, weakened immune function as well as mental disorders like anxiety and depression.

The dual nature of stress

In this chapter, I will discuss good versus harmful stress, and help you identify your stressors and how they might impact your health. I will also discuss chronic stress's profound effect on optimal wellbeing and explore the physical, emotional, and cognitive toll it can take on the body and mind.

I will focus on putting the power back into you, the blokes, by illuminating the art of stress management techniques. This chapter aims to equip you with the tools to transform stress into a catalyst for growth while safeguarding your overall health and vitality, but like the previous chapter, there is no cookie-cutter approach.

Stress affects everyone differently due to various factors, including genetics, personality, life experiences and coping mechanisms. While some individuals thrive under pressure, viewing stress as a challenge to overcome, others may find it overwhelming and debilitating.

These differences are influenced by bio-individuality, which recognises that each person's unique physiological and psychological makeup shapes their stress response. For instance, one person might experience physical symptoms such as headaches or high blood pressure, while another might struggle with emotional issues like anxiety or depression. Understanding these differences and what pain points trigger your stress response is essential for developing personalised stress management strategies that effectively address your needs and circumstances. Just like in the previous chapters, the cumulative impact of stress can significantly reduce the quality of your life and increase your risk of severe health complications.

Mick's story: A lesson in stress management

I remember facilitating a workshop for a construction company in Brisbane. Before I had time to close down my PowerPoint presentation, one of the audience members approached me. Mick was a 53-year-old senior executive in the finance department who found himself trapped in the relentless grip of chronic stress.

We spoke briefly and organised a private consultation outside his workplace so I could determine whether Mick was struggling with personal or professional stress or a blend of both. The presentation was on 'Becoming Multidimensional for Optimal Performance.' I think this was the trigger that made him act.

During the consultation, Mick spoke about the longevity of his work in the industry over the last 20 years. He had scaled the corporate ladder to satisfy his ego and salary expectations. He didn't appear consciously aware of the mounting pressures, including the long hours and constant demands, which were detrimental to his physical and emotional wellbeing.

But, like everything else, the compound effect was profound, and by the time he reached out to me, Mick was close to breaking point. The positive was that he sought help; the negative was that he hadn't addressed it years earlier, as his mindset was, 'I'll be right!'

After conducting my health audit with Mick, I could see he was close to breaking point. He was emotionally fragile and needed clarity, direction, solutions, and support. Mick's role as a finance executive meant navigating a world of intense deadlines, financial pressures, and ever-evolving market dynamics.

The perpetual state of alertness that Mick was under week after week accumulated chronic stress, which was setting off a cascade of physiological and psychological responses that impacted his health.

Mick initially ignored the common signs and systems of anxiety, including elevated blood pressure, irregular sleeping patterns and digestive issues. Due to his irregular sleep patterns and poor dietary habits, Mick had also developed a weakened immune system.

On top of that, emotionally, the chronic stress had led to persistent anxiety, a decline in his mood and difficulties concentrating in the workplace, which is why he sought my assistance. Before approaching me, Mick's mental health had begun to fray and he was consciously aware that this was affecting his professional decision-making skills as well as his personal relationships.

Things needed to change for Mick as soon as possible, and I expressed to him the urgency of creating boundaries and changing his current environment. I was honest and explained that acknowledging and discussing it wasn't enough; action and implementation would be the key ingredients to his long-term wellness. I could help, support, design, and create a structured plan for the future, but I couldn't implement the lifestyle sacrifices he needed.

After our initial health audit, I clarified that if Mick wanted to create change, it would be 100% up to him. Before he left our initial consult, I had already booked him for another session within three days. I made it quite clear that the shadow of chronic stress loomed large, casting its pervasive influence on not only his physical health but, more importantly, his mental and emotional wellbeing.

When Mick left our consultation, his deadline was 72 hours to review his current work and family environment and look at areas he could change immediately that would positively impact him mentally, emotionally and physically. When it came time to reflect on his choices, it was no coincidence that the three main areas included physical activity, nutrition and sleep.

Key ingredients: action and implementation

When Mick returned for his second consultation 72 hours later, he looked better because he had been brave enough to talk about his current situation and take ownership of what needed to change. After completing his health questionnaire online, our second session was about planning the implementation phase, and for Mick a key component of this phase was formulating some structure and time management.

Time management is a crucial component of stress for many executives I work with. For Mick, creating some structure enabled him to allocate time effectively for activities that promote wellbeing. It taught him that he needed structure around when to exercise, what to eat, when to eat and the importance of down-regulation. This, in turn, forced him to create structure around his sleep hygiene and look at strategies that he could implement in the future. In theory, the formula for him was relatively simple: allocating time to the fundamentals: exercise, nutrition and sleep, and staying accountable to it.

Mick understood the effect of compound interest. When we related this to his health, he understood that if he included some regular exercise in his weekly schedule, he would see a reduction in his stress hormones, which would also impact his mood. At the same time, a stable nutritional plan with more protein and less processed foods, along with improved water intake, would also support his physical and mental health.

Mick found that by allocating specific time to lifestyle biometrics that impacted his health, he felt less overwhelmed, and his chronic fatigue began to subside, improving his day-to-day tolerance levels.

Mick knew that not all stress was negative, and a crucial part of stress management was firstly addressing the stress, but more importantly, working out how to implement a strategy to reduce/improve the stress and learning the art of down-regulation.

Down-regulation needs to be daily, not weekly, monthly or quarterly. Like all muscles, the brain needs time to rest and recover. If you respect that stress is an inherent part of life and understand that it is a physiological response explicitly designed to mobilise the body's resources in the face of challenges, your relationship and how your body deals with and manages stress will be better off.

When the stress becomes chronic and overwhelming, as it did in Mick's situation, it can exact a toll on your health, affecting both your mind and your body in profound ways, which I have witnessed first-hand with many of my clients. My number one piece of advice is to act now or suffer later. It would be best if you were accountable for your stress management techniques and like the other dimensions, stay consistent.

ACTIVITY

REFLECTING ON YOUR STRESS AND WELLBEING

Take a moment to reflect on how stress impacts you. Use this activity to identify specific triggers and explore ways to minimise them, helping you gain insight into both the positive and negative effects of stress on your emotional, cognitive and physical health.

Complete these steps:

1. Consider the stress you encounter and assess its impact on your wellbeing, both positive (good stress) and negative (bad stress).

2. Consider how you feel emotionally, cognitively and physically.

3. Write a few points down.

4. What were the triggers that led to this stress response?

5. How can you minimise or reduce these stressors in your life?

Good stress versus bad stress

Like everything in life, there is always good and evil; when it comes to stress, we must respect and embrace this attitude. Good or positive stress is typically characterised by short-term challenges that motivate and energise you. This might drive your achievements, growth and resilience for some of you. On the contrary, distress is bad stress or negative stress, which is typically chronic and accompanied by feelings of anxiety, overwhelm and a sense of helplessness, similar to the signs and symptoms Mick suffered. I have seen this repeatedly when dealing with corporate types and it is the body's response to harmful stress.

Stress can lead to a cascade of physiological and psychological consequences if prolonged. Just remember that any word that describes something as 'chronic' highlights its level of importance and this is mainly the case when we refer to harmful stress. Typically, this is characterised by someone who is suffering from a prolonged and unrelenting state of psychological and physiological stress and for me, this poses a significant threat to one's overall health and wellbeing.

Primary risk of chronic stress

Medical research suggests that up to 90% of illnesses and diseases are linked to stress (*Institute of Functional Medicine* 2024). Chronic stress, in particular, poses a significant risk to cardiovascular health. I have observed this, especially in executives facing relentless pressures in the corporate world. These constant demands lead to ongoing surges in stress hormones, particularly cortisol, which can raise blood pressure, heart rate and inflammation levels.

Over time, these physical responses to stress become silent but severe contributors to the risk of hypertension, coronary artery disease and other cardiovascular issues. Left unchecked, these conditions can develop into life-threatening diseases. This is especially concerning, as cardiovascular disease—the leading cause of death in men—is almost entirely preventable with proper management of stress and lifestyle.

Another chronic stress response is its effect on your immune system, a critical line of defence against illnesses, which becomes compromised in the face of chronic stress. Again, this is highlighted with executives grappling with persistent anxiety, finding themselves more susceptible to infections due to their weakened immune responses, diminishing their ability to fend off common illnesses. I cannot overstate the importance of good sleep hygiene, regular exercise, and proper nutrition to support a strong immune system. Supplementation can also play a role, particularly in addressing poor eating habits, with options like vitamin D, multivitamins, ashwagandha, and more.

The ripple effect on hormonal and mental health

Hormonal imbalance is another symptom of chronic stress, which is caused by elevated cortisol levels. This can also disrupt the delicate balance of other hormones, including testosterone, which will affect your sex life, not to mention erectile dysfunction—and nobody wants that. Therefore, the impact on hormonal health not only affects personal relationships but can also have broader implications for a man's sense of wellbeing and self-esteem, which leads me to my fourth primary health risk, mental health.

Mental health bears a heavy burden under the weight of chronic stress for male corporate executives. The relentless demands of leadership roles can contribute to elevated levels of anxiety and depression. Persistent stress is associated with cognitive impairments, including difficulties with concentration, memory and decision-making. The toll on mental health is not only detrimental to individual executives but can also affect the overall dynamics and productivity of the workplace.

Another chronic stress response in Mick was gut health and digestive system disruptions. Typically, irritable bowel syndrome (IBS) and digestive disorders often surface because of prolonged stress. It then becomes a snowball effect as these physical manifestations of stress not only contribute to discomfort but also impact nutritional health, creating a cycle of physical and mental distress.

Finally, following the previous chapter, poor sleep is also related to chronic stress, perpetuating a cycle of fatigue and heightened stress levels. Mick had terrible sleeping patterns because he found it difficult to fall asleep. He would wake up multiple times during the night and found it extremely difficult to achieve restorative sleep. He couldn't down-regulate.

The importance of addressing chronic stress early

If you are reading this chapter and can relate to Mick's situation, you need to address the cause of your chronic stress. Typically, whatever the cause or causes of chronic stress, it is essential to understand how to manage it. It usually requires a multifaceted approach, encompassing lifestyle changes and other coping strategies and, when necessary, professional help.

As I have highlighted in previous chapters, the implementation is tricky. The most challenging part was when Mick required professional intervention (lifestyle medicine). I was fortunate and grateful that I could assist him on his road to optimal health. I was not the cure, and our work together wasn't the end, but it was undoubtedly a great start.

On a personal level, if you are unwilling to invest in your health and wellbeing and seek professional help, then at least begin with regular physical activity, including some mindfulness practices and watch what you eat. I also encourage social connectivity, which you will read more about in Chapter 9, and support from peers, family, friends and work colleagues.

Recognising and actively addressing chronic stress will improve your physical and mental wellbeing and enhance your resilience to life's challenges.

Techniques to minimise stress

You don't need medication; you need meditation

For Mick, the first stage was taking ownership and identifying the lifestyle factors causing his chronic stress. His work landscape was a key contributor. Still, the secondary factors—no exercise, poor dietary habits, and disrupted sleep—had the most significant impact on his health and wellbeing.

Recognising the signs of stress and, more importantly, implementing effective coping strategies are pivotal for mitigating stress's negative impact on overall health. Many people struggle with this in isolation. Many people think these signs and symptoms will pass or dissipate, but there is no short-term solution if you aren't willing to change your environment.

When clients feel anxious or stressed, my first advice is to implement regular physical activity into their daily routines. For me, exercise is non-negotiable, but typically, when executives have periods of late nights and long days, combined with a lack of sleep and poor nutritional habits, lacing up their runners is the last thing they want to do. Yet, it is the best and cheapest form of medicine. When Mick approached me, he was not exercising at all as he had 'no time.' Therefore, his initial lifestyle medicine was getting him to acknowledge that he needed to change and start exercising.

Once he established a routine, he gradually increased his intensity, duration and frequency. The key was to identify first, then design and finally implement an exercise plan that Mick could sustain, regardless of his work schedule/commitments.

I remember setting up Mick's baseline program when we started. It was only 20 minutes, including an eight-minute brisk walk and a bodyweight circuit. His walking pace had to be honest, and his heart rate had to increase. After eight minutes, he had to do five step-ups on a park bench on each leg, then 10 push-ups, 10 squats, 10 bodyweight dips, five lunges on each leg, 15 sit-ups, 10 torso rotations and then finish with a plank for as long as he could. He could then rest for two minutes before repeating it.

It was short and challenging for Mick, yet achievable in only 20 minutes. Over time, the aim would be to increase his repetitions, lengthen his cardio from eight to 15 minutes (Zone 2) and then get Mick from walking to jogging when he started feeling fitter and more robust.

As I mentioned in Chapter 5, exercise has many benefits. Still, for Mick and many of my clients, regular exercise is also a potent stress reliever, as it stimulates the release of endorphins, which we know are the body's natural mood enhancers.

Another stress response Mick needed to address was slowing his mind down. His daily schedule was always busy, in and out of meetings, on conference calls and dealing with staff issues and daily challenges in the construction industry.

So, to improve his sleeping habits, cognitive function and clarity, we worked on a few mindfulness practices. I would get Mick to practice a few meditation techniques in the morning. While at work, I'd call Mick to focus on breathing exercises and then at night, I encouraged Mick to journal to slow his mind down. Over time, these three easy techniques had a profound effect on enhancing Mick's emotional resilience.

We also looked at strategies to establish and maintain a healthy work-life balance to support Mick's ongoing mental health. So, if you can identify with Mick and the struggles he encountered due to chronic work stress, write down a few things you need to change to minimise your 'bad stressors.' Reflect on your work pressures, time management, exercise frequency, nutritional habits, sleep hygiene and mental health. Typically, during my initial health audit, I ask all my clients to complete a personalised scorecard (see below), self-evaluating their health to identify potential stressors.

Personalised score cards

Exercise frequency (number of weekly sessions)

(Nil   1   2   3   4   5   6   7)

Hours sleep per night

(4—6   6.5—8   8.5+)

Eating habits

(Poor   Average   Good   Excellent)

Hydration platform (daily water consumption)

(.5 L   1 L   1.5   2 L   2.5 L)

Social connectivity

(Nil   Daily   Weekly   Fortnightly   Monthly)

Regular holidays

(Nil   Monthly   Quarterly   Yearly)

Once you have reviewed the personalised scorecard, you can identify which external factors have the most significant impact on your stress levels. You can then actively design a tailored plan to suit your stressors and test and measure the effect of 'lifestyle medicine' on your stress levels. Remember, if you measure, you can manage.

Lifestyle strategies to reduce stress might include one or more of the following:

1. **Establishing clear boundaries:**
   - Set clear boundaries between work and personal life to prevent burnout. Avoid bringing work-related stressors into personal time.
   - Use technology tools to set specific times for work-related communications and notifications.

2. **Implementing regular exercise:**

   Incorporate regular physical activity into your routine to alleviate stress. Exercise releases endorphins, natural mood boosters and reduces levels of the body's stress hormone cortisol.

3. **Healthy diet:**
   - Monitor your food consumption and, where possible, maintain a diet rich in fruits, vegetables, lean protein and whole grains.
   - Be consciously aware of the amount of caffeine, sugar and processed foods you consume, as they all exacerbate stress.

4. **Adequate sleep:**
   - Ensure you get enough sleep each night by establishing a regular sleep routine and optimum sleep environment, in particular, avoiding screens before bed.
   - The key to sleep is slowing the brain down and allowing it time to recover, which is essential for physical and mental recovery.

5. Mindfulness and relaxation techniques:

- Practice mindfulness and relaxation techniques, such as meditation, deep-breathing exercises or progressive muscle relaxation.

- Consider incorporating mindfulness apps or wellness programs into your daily routines.

6. Time management and prioritisation:

- Focus on high-impact activities.

- Delegate responsibilities, when possible, to avoid becoming overwhelmed by an excessive workload.

7. Effective communication:

- Foster open communication within the workplace to address concerns and challenges before the stress becomes chronic (ask Mick). Encourage a supportive and collaborative work environment.

- Develop strong interpersonal skills to navigate complex professional relationships and reduce interpersonal stress.

8. Build a support system:

- Cultivate a robust support system, both within and outside the workplace. Establishing meaningful connections with colleagues and friends can provide emotional support.

- Consider seeking guidance from other health professionals or engaging your employee assistance program to help minimise stress.

Mick reached a turning point where he decided to take control of his wellbeing. Without seeking help, he knew he was at risk of becoming another statistic in the corporate world, where burnout and health issues are prevalent.

Through his concerted efforts, Mick experienced a remarkable transformation. Physically, his blood pressure stabilised and his digestive issues dissipated. Emotionally, he reported reduced anxiety levels, improved mood and enhanced concentration. The positive changes in his lifestyle not only alleviated the immediate effects of chronic stress but also positioned him on a trajectory toward sustained wellbeing.

When you have a client like Mick who acknowledges his problem but wants to improve his situation, my role as an executive health coach is rewarding.

Mick's journey is a testament to the transformative power of holistic wellbeing practices and 'lifestyle medicine' in overcoming chronic stress, which is why I love this industry. You don't need medication to minimise your chronic stress; you need consistent 'lifestyle' strategies that suit you. Mick is living proof of this by taking control of his lifestyle, implementing boundaries and cultivating healthy habits.

Mick's case underscores the importance of recognising the signs of chronic stress and actively pursuing a comprehensive approach to wellbeing to safeguard one's health in the demanding landscape of corporate leadership.

By adopting lifestyle stress-reduction techniques, fostering a supportive social network and being proactive about overall wellbeing, you can navigate the challenges of stress and cultivate resilience in the face of life's adversities. This is why I emphasise the importance of being 'multidimensional' and taking a comprehensive approach to managing stress for long-term health optimisation.

Five-step blueprint for reducing stress

Step 1: Identify your stress triggers

The first step in managing stress is understanding what causes it. Identify the sources of your stress, whether related to work, relationships, health, finances or other areas of your life. Keep a stress journal to track your triggers, how you respond and how these stressors affect your mood and physical state. Awareness of your stressors is crucial for developing effective coping strategies.

Step 2: Develop healthy coping strategies

Once you've identified your stress triggers, develop healthy coping strategies. This may include physical activities like exercise, which can help reduce stress hormones and boost endorphins. Incorporate relaxation techniques such as deep breathing, meditation or progressive muscle relaxation to calm your mind. Engaging in hobbies, spending time in nature or connecting with friends and family can also help alleviate stress.

Step 3: Prioritise time management and organisation

Poor time management and disorganisation can contribute significantly to stress. Create a daily or weekly plan to manage your tasks and responsibilities effectively. Prioritise your to-do list by focusing on the most critical tasks and breaking larger tasks into smaller, manageable steps. Use tools like planners, apps or digital calendars to keep track of deadlines and commitments. Set boundaries around your time to avoid overcommitting and ensure you allocate time for self-care.

Step 4: Practice mindfulness and stay present

Mindfulness involves staying present and fully engaged in the current moment, which can help reduce anxiety about the past or future. Incorporate mindfulness practices into your daily routine, such as mindful breathing, meditation or simply focusing on your surroundings. Mindfulness helps you become more aware of your thoughts and emotions, allowing you to respond to stress more calmly and deliberately.

Step 5: Take care of your physical health

Your physical health is intricately linked to your ability to manage stress. Sleep well, eat a balanced diet, stay hydrated and exercise regularly. Limit caffeine, alcohol and sugar, as these can increase anxiety and disrupt sleep. Adequate rest, proper nutrition and regular physical activity support your body's resilience to stress, helping you feel more balanced and better equipped to manage life's challenges.

By following this five-step blueprint, you can create a structured approach to reducing stress, enhancing your ability to cope with challenges and improving your overall wellbeing. Consistent practice of these steps will help you build resilience, maintain a calm mindset and navigate stressful situations more effectively.

What, how, when: the core trio for reducing stress

1. What:

- Identify your stress management goals: Start by defining your goals for stress reduction. Clear goals will guide your actions and help you measure progress.

- Stress management goals: What specific aspects of stress do you want to address? This might include reducing overall stress levels, managing stress more effectively in particular situations (for example, at work or home) or improving emotional resilience.

2. How:

- Implement effective stress reduction strategies: Determine how you will achieve your stress management goals. This involves choosing and applying specific techniques and strategies that work for you.
- Stress reduction techniques: How will you manage stress? Adopt a mix of strategies such as:
    - Physical activity: Regular exercise like walking, yoga or strength training.
    - Relaxation practices: Incorporate deep breathing, meditation or progressive muscle relaxation into your routine.
    - Time management: Use tools like planners or apps to organise tasks and set priorities.
    - Mindfulness: Practice mindfulness techniques to stay present and reduce anxiety about the future or past.
- Healthy lifestyle choices: Maintain good sleep hygiene, enjoy a balanced diet and stay hydrated.

3. When:

- Schedule and integrate stress management practices: Specify when you will practice your stress reduction strategies to ensure they become a routine.
- Stress management schedule: When will you incorporate these practices into your daily or weekly routine? For example:
    - Daily: Set aside 10–15 minutes each morning for mindfulness or meditation and integrate short periods of physical activity throughout your day.
    - Weekly: Plan regular exercise sessions, such as three times a week and allocate time for relaxation or hobbies on weekends.
    - As needed: Use stress management techniques during particularly stressful situations or when you notice increased stress.

Take the first step towards lasting wellbeing: create your personalised stress reduction plan

You can build a structured, sustainable plan that seamlessly integrates effective techniques into your daily life by specifying the core trio of 'what, how and when' of stress reduction. This clear formula allows you to proactively identify and tackle stress triggers, using tailored strategies that suit your unique needs and lifestyle. By reducing stress consistently and effectively, you are enhancing your immediate wellbeing and building resilience that prepares you for future challenges. Start exploring your approach to stress today—taking small, manageable steps to transform how you respond to life's pressures can lead to a healthier, more balanced you.

WRITE DOWN YOUR PLAN HERE:

What:

_____
_____
_____
_____
_____
_____

How:

_____
_____
_____
_____
_____
_____

When:

_____
_____
_____
_____
_____
_____

CHAPTER 9

Social connectivity

No man is an island. No man stands alone.

—John Donne

The value of social connections for health and wellbeing

Many of us take social connections for granted. Yet, a large body of research shows that social isolation and loneliness have a severe impact on physical and mental health, quality of life and longevity. As blokes, we have 'mates,' but sometimes, we are left vulnerable because of the level of connectedness in our friendships.

From the outside, we have all the resources to stay socially connected with access to many social media platforms. Yet, the statistics show that meaningful social contact has declined across all age groups in Australia for decades.

In this chapter, I will explore the profound impact of social interaction on mental, emotional and physical health. I will discuss the devastating effects of social isolation and loneliness. I will unravel the compelling reasons why cultivating social connections is not merely a luxury but a necessity for optimal health. From the camaraderie forged in sporting clubs to the shared purpose within organisations, I will discuss the transformative power of groups in enhancing social connectivity.

In the business world, there is a lot of data and evidence about the success of building a great culture and how it translates to better profit margins and a happier and healthier workforce. The simple fact is the happier the employee, the more motivated the employee. So, during this chapter, I will encourage you to find your 'elite performance team members' and then harness the art of positive social connectivity.

This chapter is the roadmap, providing insights and practical strategies to weave the vital thread of connection into the lives of men, starting with the *Blokes Inc. Play a Bigger Game* community, fostering a robust foundation for wellbeing and resilience moving forward.

Questions for reflection

Ask yourself these questions:

- Do you feel socially connected?
- Who are your 'elite team members' in life?
- Think of a sports team or a work team you were part of? What made it successful?

Mt Eliza friendships #aussiecrawl

I grew up on the Mornington Peninsula in a bayside suburb called Mt Eliza. At the time, I took it for granted; however, looking back, I was fortunate enough to go to Peninsula Grammar School from age five until I completed my final year of study as an 18-year-old.

I have so many fond memories of growing up in Mt Eliza and the older I get, the better the recollections become. Peninsula was a private boys' school during my school days, but in 1994 it became co-educational. The friendships I made at school, both a year below and a year above, were solid. Many are still strong today, which speaks volumes of the type of friendship we created throughout my schooling.

Growing up in a small town, everyone knew each other and at times, their private lives cross-pollinated over the years. But one thing that remained tight was our loyalty to our friendships and our mates.

When I arrived in London as a 23-year-old who had been travelling abroad for three months this camaraderie was highlighted. Low on cash flow, I had organised to stay with a few mates from school until I found a job and an income.

In my backpacking days, we didn't have the luxury of mobile phones, so any form of communication was infrequent and we only used email at internet cafes. I remember that before I left Spain, I received an email from my one of my best mates, Silly who had been based in London for a year or so and it was where I would stay until I got sorted.

The email was his directions to the shared accommodation in Bayswater, which meant getting from Heathrow airport to Baywater using the Underground and at the time the directions seemed brief and rough. The first commute was straightforward: get on the London underground and head from Heathrow Airport to Bayswater Station using the Tube.

I remember thinking it was a Tuesday morning, so most people Silly shared the accommodation with would be at work, including himself. As I exited the train doors to the familiar train station audio announcement of *mind the gap*, my first commute was complete; now it was time to find the house…

Walking along Bayswater Road from the station, I could hear this gentle bass music gradually getting louder and louder. *Doof, doof, doof, doof.*

I approached the traffic lights exactly where I was supposed to be. Silly had explained the apartment was on the corner of Bayswater Road and Paddington Palace, levels one to three.

I looked up and saw nothing resembling a lovely inner-city apartment with planter boxes; all I saw was what looked like a day club. I put my backpack down, found the piece of paper with the correct address, checked the number on the paper, looked at the apartment, rechecked the number and thought, *surely not*. I walked across the road with trepidation and looked up to people smoking out the windows.

'TT,' I heard someone yell. 'TT's here! Come up! Hey, someone let TT in.'

WTF, I thought. *Tuesday 11.00 am*?

As I walked up the stairs, the music was loud. The kitchen featured a smoke machine, and a DJ was set up in the lounge room. Bodies and people were everywhere.

'Welcome, mate. A few of us are just having a few drinks while the others are at work. You will sleep upstairs on the top level with Hilly and Silly, so put your backpack up there, they are both at work.'

As I headed up the stairs, I couldn't believe it; it felt like I was back in Mt Eliza, so many familiar faces. It was like I had my own welcoming committee, with smiles, hugs and kisses, although overwhelming. I hadn't seen many of these people for years, but the friendships we established throughout our school days stood the test of time. It was like we had seen each other yesterday. Connecting with people who understand, value and support my true sense of social connection!

Seeing these school friends felt like stepping back in time, surrounded by familiar faces and the warmth of old friendships that had not faded with the years. These connections reminded me of the power of genuine social bonds—ones that make you feel understood, valued and genuinely connected.

Link between isolation, loneliness and mortality

In earlier chapters, I discussed the impact poor nutrition and inactivity have on longevity. In this chapter, you will see the correlation between social isolation, loneliness and mortality.

As an executive health coach, I often work with clients who have lost their social connectivity, predominantly due to their work commitments. These clients are 100% engaged in their work tasks, deadlines, and KPIs but fail to invest in their relationships with friends and family.

Typically, I define these people as being one-dimensional. They have surface-level conversations in the office but no meaningful conversations. Part of my support role as a coach is listening, providing support, suggesting advice, encouraging alternatives and then reframing situations or scenarios for my clients. Often, they need a sounding board as they don't feel comfortable sharing their personal/professional issues with loved ones, family members or fellow employees, but they know they need social engagement.

Case study: Peter

I remember a client of mine, Peter, a 51-year-old corporate executive who had spent most of his career climbing the corporate ladder since entering the workforce. After years of working in the Melbourne and Sydney offices, Peter was offered a promotion, which involved relocating to Hong Kong.

Here is Peter's first email to me:

> Subject: Seeking guidance for a holistic wellness journey
>
> Dear Tory,
>
> I hope this email finds you well.
>
> My name is Peter and I enjoyed attending one of your wellness presentations on becoming 'multidimensional' many years ago. I was genuinely inspired by your style and the comprehensive approach you advocated for achieving overall wellbeing. I need more than just a physical reboot at this point in my life. I seek your expertise, knowledge, advice and motivation to help guide me on a holistic wellness journey. Your presentation resonated deeply with me and with your guidance, I can make meaningful and lasting changes in my life and hopefully dig myself out of my current fog.
>
> I would appreciate any advice or resources you can provide to help me get started. Whether it be one-on-one consultations, coaching or any other support, I am eager to learn and commit to improving my health and wellbeing on all levels. My issue is that I am no longer based in Melbourne; I have moved to Hong Kong.
>
> Thank you very much for your time and consideration. I look forward to working with you and benefiting from your invaluable expertise.
>
> Warm regards,
>
> Peter

Having scrutinised Peter's email, I organised a Zoom consultation to provide direction.

During this initial consultation, Peter and I discussed his move to Hong Kong, his lack of connection outside the workplace and look at what a typical day looked like compared to his weekend activities/engagements. I referenced the adverse effects of a lack of social connection to see if that resonated with him, but his body language remained fairly neutral.

Peter thought that burying himself in his work commitments would improve things or justify why he felt so bad. Yet, over time, his sense of loneliness never changed. He always felt run down, which he thought was a response to his lack of sleep.

Emotionally and cognitively, he also highlighted that his sense of happiness was below average and that his ability to focus was deteriorating. He was becoming disengaged personally and professionally.

With over 20 years of direct experience working with people and observing their responses, I'm not surprised by studies showing that humans are inherently social creatures. When deprived of meaningful social interactions, various aspects of wellbeing can suffer. For Peter, this lack of social connection had a particularly profound impact on his health.

Initially, Peter said he was excited about the professional opportunity. However, he moved without fully considering its impact on his social connections and, subsequently, his overall wellbeing.

Upon relocating, Peter was in a new city, far away from friends and family. His demanding job left little time for socialising and his few interactions were limited to office settings. Weekends were often spent catching up on work or exploring the new city alone.

Over time, the lack of social connections took a toll on Peter's mental and physical health and that was when he connected with me. When Peter reached out, he was disillusioned and confused. He knew something was wrong but couldn't quite identify it.

Due to Peter's location, we spent several hours on Zoom, talking about his workload, travel commitments, and the stress he felt about his work commitments versus the stress directly related to his lifestyle (living away from family and friends).

I suggested Peter get his blood work done to ensure his physical health was sound. This would allow me to review his blood profile and see if there were any 'outliers' or disease markers.

Peter's other physiological symptoms were standard for any corporate executive working 60-plus hours per week. Poor sleep hygiene, weight gain, elevated levels of cortisol, excessive alcohol intake and zero exercise. All of which could lead to lifestyle diseases if untreated.

Yet, the lack of social connectivity impacting Peter's physical and emotional health. In Melbourne, Peter would frequently meet with his mates, go for a bike ride along Beach Road and grab coffee before starting his day. Friday after work, there was always an opportunity to grab a beer or go to the footy (AFL) with his mates on the weekend.

For many executives, these social activities are a simple 'stress buster,' considerably improving their emotional health. Yet, Peter took this for granted. He had done it for years; however, since his relocation, he had no morning routine. The culture of after-work drinks or going to a sporting event didn't exist in Hong Kong, or if it did Peter's lack of connection meant he wasn't aware of it. He just buried himself in his role, stayed in the office late and rinsed and repeated day in and day out.

Over the years, I have worked with plenty of executives whose sole focus has been on their careers. They were willing to sacrifice anything to climb the corporate ladder to increase their net worth. I witnessed and worked with it firsthand. The weight gain, the stress, the infidelity, the destructive behaviour and the lack of social connection all have a profound effect on one's physical and mental health.

Peter loved his work and the company he worked for, but he started to get resentful, blaming everything negative in his life on his work environment—the lack of downtime, the workload, the constant pressure to meet deadlines, the meetings—but it was so much deeper than this. Thankfully, this was when Peter decided to contact me searching for answers—and we found the answer!

Negative effects of a lack of social connection

Numerous studies have shown that there is an increased risk of several health issues that are related to a lack of social connectivity (Holt-Lunstad et al 2015). Typically, the first sign is poor physical health.

Chronic social isolation has been linked to a weakened immune system, making individuals more susceptible to illnesses and infections. This lack of social connection is also associated with an increased risk of cardiovascular problems such as high blood pressure and heart disease. Strong social ties have a protective effect on heart health; and in Peter's case, this was obvious. Living and working in Melbourne, he enjoyed weekly road cycling sessions followed by a caffeine hit. In Hong Kong, road cycling was impossible.

In many cases, the lack of social connectivity leads to sleep disturbances, which tend to be a blend of the emotional and psychological effects of loneliness. In Peter's circumstance, the absence of a social support network amplified his emotional distress. Peter's original email to me was a call for help as he found it difficult to cope with life's difficulties, which were more challenging because he felt he had no one to share the burden with or seek advice from. For some people, this lack of connection/trust and the absence of regular social interactions can lead to feelings of emptiness and sadness, leading to anxiety.

In more extreme circumstances, it can contribute to a state of depression. Peter talked about how his cognitive health was on the decline. More recently, research has found that social isolation may contribute to an increased risk of developing Alzheimer's disease and other forms of dementia (Langa 2018). Typically, these cases presented when there were no social interactions to stimulate cognitive function and the absence of such stimulation accelerated cognitive decline. In Peter's case, I think the fatigue, lack of sleep and stress affected his mental functioning.

Peter and I picked apart these adverse effects concerning his lack of social connectivity to see how many were relevant to him.

Without familiar faces and a support system, Peter felt isolated and lonely. The absence of social interactions outside of work contributed to his sense of detachment and melancholy.

I could see his expression change when he spoke about his fond memories of cycling before work and the banter his cycling group would have at the coffee shop afterwards. 'Those were the days,' he repeatedly said.

Peter also articulated that the pressure of his executive role, combined with his relocation and the lack of social support, led to heightened stress levels and increased anxiety and the only way he was dealing with this was by working more.

Peter admitted that he was constantly on edge, struggling to find a healthy work-life balance. Even on weekends, he struggled to switch off and focus on rest and recovery. He could not down-regulate. His ego was now in full swing, his cortisol levels (stress hormone) were high and the emotional strain and stress translated to poor sleep quality.

The nights were restless, and he often woke up feeling fatigued, which impacted his ability to perform optimally at work. His morning rituals were the caffeine shot, the cold shower, and then straight-on task—quite a contrast to a ride down Beach Road with his mates.

But instead of looking at avenues to improve his energy levels through good nutrition and a sound exercise plan, he consumed more caffeine and then self-medicated after work with wine before bed. Every day, Peter woke up tired and weary, leading to a sedentary lifestyle and stress, which contributed to his weight gain and a decline in overall physical fitness.

Thankfully, Peter's blood profile showed no elevated disease markers. He had a balanced cholesterol score, normal glucose levels, and healthy liver and kidney function, which was pleasing. Fortunately, the key indicators of any chronic condition, such as white and red blood cell counts, haemoglobin levels, and inflammatory markers like C-reactive protein, were all within the standard reference ranges.

So, after identifying all the negative aspects of Peter's work environment, our immediate plan was to inject positivity into his daily routine. My plan involved working closely with Peter via Zoom twice weekly to reinforce that we needed to focus on several lifestyle factors to help his overall wellbeing.

An essential component included taking proactive steps to rebuild Peter's social connections outside the workplace. He acknowledged that his success at work shouldn't come at the expense of his mental and physical health, which was significantly impacting his function inside and outside of the workplace. This caused self-doubt; he blamed his job and resented the promotion and the relocation.

No different to nutrition, exercise and stress, everyone has different drivers that add or subtract value to our overall wellbeing, so we mustn't neglect our friends, family and ability to stay connected. Remember, we all need a *team* that supports us.

More on Peter later…

> There is no such thing as a self-made man. You will reach your goal with the help of others.
>
> —George Shinn

Withdrawal: a double-edged sword in depression

When I transitioned from health into hospitability, which quickly became a failure, I withdrew from all my close friends and family. I was embarrassed and ashamed of my professional situation. The longer my professional crisis lasted, the more I withdrew; I went away from everything I talked and preached about to executives for 10 years prior. I neglected my health, my family, my lifestyle and my friends.

In 2019, my wife and I moved to the beautiful coastal town of Byron Bay in Northern New South Wales. Before meeting each other, we had both spent times living and working abroad, but aside from those experiences, we had each lived in Victoria our entire lives.

When we lived in Victoria, we would regularly holiday in Byron Bay and ask ourselves the same question, 'Could we live here?' Generally, the answer was no; I had created and established a personal training and corporate health business in Melbourne, and Fi had a great corporate job. We also had our families and friends that we knew we'd miss.

After 20 years in the health space, I was constantly looking for more and I would continually ask myself what I could do outside of the health and fitness industry. How could I create wealth and enjoy a better lifestyle for our young family? This internal dialogue started well before I was married, but at that stage, I was comfortable; I had a team of trainers, a few significant corporate contracts and money in the bank.

I had previously started a mobile juice company called Liquid Hit and I bought and sold a group exercise business called GET, which stands for Group Exercise Therapy. I had help design, test and manufacture an isotonic sports drink, LFE Isotonic. Fi and I also bought and sold an online activewear company, Active Style. She had also developed an app called Mumafit, which targeted pre- and post-pregnancy women. So, we couldn't be classified as lazy! We both had a strong work ethic and a desire to succeed and live our desired life.

My desire for change grew as our family grew; I had been counting reps, talking diet and motivating the masses for over 20 years. Through my core business, I was fortunate that I had many affluent clients, but this was a curse because at the same time I aspired for their lifestyle (maybe just a fraction of their wealth). Many were self-made, successful business people involved in retail, property, financial services and hospitality.

As time continued to pass, my thirst for change increased until I finally started speaking to one of my clients, who had founded a hospitality franchise. Sure, the word 'franchise' should have been a red flag, but I had known the founder for over five years, personally and professionally. Like many other franchisees, my mentality was that it wouldn't happen to me; this business/franchise was a foolproof business that was very successful in Melbourne.

As I said, I knew the founder and another client was an early investor. I also learned about a few store owners winning the financial lottery with this business, which excited me. I decided I wanted to be a part of it.

You are probably asking, *why the franchise?* And *why Byron Bay?* Both very valid questions, but for me, it ticked two boxes: Firstly, the franchise model allowed for consistency, training, setup, staffing, and so forth. Secondly, there was nothing like this product in Byron Bay and I thought Byron Bay needed this quality product. Anyway, the discussions started, my wife agreed to relocate and I thought now was the time for a career change! What a disaster this was. As soon as I committed to not one but two franchises, the train wreck began.

Four weeks after opening, we realised the shop fitter (recommended by the franchisor) hadn't paid the local tradies even though we had paid him. As a new family in town, we couldn't afford a bad reputation as our kids had just started at the local primary school, so we paid each tradie directly, effectively double-dipping.

So, before the doors were even open, we were negative $85,000. To make matters worse, the same shopfitter had committed to completing our second store, 45 minutes north at a growing part of the Gold Coast, Palm Beach, straight after completing Byron Bay.

Before we had become aware of the shopfitter shortfall, we had already committed $100,000 to the Palm Beach build. It was too late to find out and the alarm bells rang. As a sign of this human personality, I confronted him and he liquidated the business and walked off the job.

Now we were down $185,000! Thinking things couldn't get worse, they did.

To complete the second store's construction, I sold 50% of the business to a person from Melbourne who told me a good story when I was at my most vulnerable. What a disaster!

This guy was a human with no moral compass, and not only did he destroy the business reputation, but he also nearly destroyed my wife with his verbal assault, not to mention physically assaulting me and sexual harassment to staff and Uber drivers. More unpaid debts followed, and the list goes on. It is hard to believe that these types of people exist!

From 2019 until July 2023, I felt like I was constantly being pushed into the UFC ring. Each time I'd enter the Octagon, I'd tap out, but the judge would ignore my decision.

Withdrawing from friends and family

To give you an idea of how I felt day in and day out is hard for me to articulate. Everything I had preached for 20 years; I was doing the opposite. I wasn't eating well. I was drinking too much alcohol. I wasn't exercising, and I withdrew from my friends and family. I'd turn up to work smiling at customers, but internally, I was crying.

I knew every day I turned on the lights, we were losing money. I felt like I was slowly drowning. I could see the lifeguards, but they couldn't see me. This feeling wasn't just for days, weeks or months. It was years!

Learning to share the burden

The experience was challenging to articulate, so I withdrew from my core group of mates. I had numerous missed calls, voicemails and

WhatsApp messages, but I had little value to offer, so I ignored the calls. But mates are mates and they always have your back. I remember two great mates flying up for a weekend to offer support.

I internally knew that they couldn't solve my business problems, but the fact that they provided support and an ear to listen gave me hope. I remember one of my good mates, Silly, said a problem shared is a problem halved. I wish I had reached out a little earlier.

So, if you have something internally causing you stress, I encourage you to share your thoughts, talk about it and be open and honest to those who are there to listen or return the favour to another friend. You don't need a big team, but you need to know that someone has your back in the good and bad times. Remember, you are not alone; many people deal with similar stressors/experiences. Please drop your ego and share.

Never let the present dictate your future; stay true to your gut feelings, stay strong and find a way.

An often-quoted quote by Albert Einstein, Benjamin Franklin or others who probably never said it is that 'insanity may be defined as doing the same thing over and over and expecting different results.' This was me, 110%.

Every day, I went to work looking for the answer, hoping the circumstances would change and every day, my wife had the same answer and was getting extremely frustrated with me. Fi is exceptionally bright and loves spreadsheets and numbers; she continually told me to close the doors, but that was easier said than done.

We had already invested and lost most of our finances, and I wasn't willing to go down without a fight. What did I learn? I learnt that hospitality is hard, but it becomes even harder when you attempt to trade through two years of COVID-19 in a tourist town.

We had supply agreements, bank finance and supplier debt. The only way to get out without digging deeper into debt was to sell it. After four years, was it worth anything? Not really, but the upside was that I could sell the business without the franchise, which eventually is what we did.

I worked my last shift at the end of June 2023. I walked out much poorer financially but perhaps one day richer for the experience…

To say the entire experience strained our marriage and family would be an understatement and a disservice. However, we are still together. Sure, the kids witnessed and heard more than they should, but hopefully, they were young enough to forget.

The real question is, how did I survive? How did our marriage survive? I honestly think about this a lot, but without my mates, a strong work ethic, a desire to help my family and a patient wife, I know I wouldn't have.

So, if you are in a similar situation, I encourage you to be open, transparent, vulnerable and brave enough to ask for help and, at the very least, communicate with others. It's the hardest thing to do, but remember, a problem shared is a problem halved and connecting with people who understand you, value you and support you is the true sense of social connection.

I honestly can't thank my mates enough!

Five-step blueprint for improving social connectivity

Step 1: Assess your current social network

Start by evaluating your existing social connections. Identify key relationships, including family, friends, colleagues and community members. Reflect on the quality and frequency of your interactions with these people. Assess areas where you feel connected and places where you might want to build or improve relationships. Understanding your current social landscape will help you pinpoint opportunities for enhancement.

Step 2: Set clear social connectivity goals

Define specific goals for improving your social connectivity. These goals should align with your personal and professional aspirations. For example, you might aim to strengthen existing relationships, make new friends, expand your professional network or become more involved in community activities. Use the SMART criteria (Specific, Measurable, Achievable, Relevant, Time-bound) to set clear, actionable objectives.

Step 3: Develop a strategy for building and maintaining connections

Create a strategic plan for enhancing your social connectivity. This plan should include practical steps for reaching your goals and maintaining relationships.

- Networking: Attend social events, join clubs or groups related to your interests and participate in community activities to meet new people.
- Communication: Regularly contact friends and family through calls, texts or social media. Schedule catchups or check-ins to maintain and strengthen relationships.

- Support: Offer support and help to others when needed and be open to receiving support. This reciprocity fosters more robust and more meaningful connections.

Step 4: Integrate social activities into your routine

Incorporate social activities into your daily or weekly routine to make them a regular part of your life. Schedule time for social interactions just as you would for work or personal commitments.

- Daily: Engage in small, everyday social interactions, such as chatting with colleagues or neighbours.
- Weekly: Plan regular activities, such as family dinners, friend meetups or professional networking events.
- Monthly: Attend more significant social events, participate in community gatherings or volunteer for local causes.

Step 5: Reflect and adjust your approach

Review and assess the effectiveness of your social connectivity efforts regularly. Reflect on your progress towards your goals and the quality of your relationships. Consider what is working well and what might need adjustment. If necessary, solicit feedback from trusted friends or mentors and be open to adapting your strategies to meet your social connectivity objectives better.

Back to Peter...

Following this five-step blueprint, you can systematically enhance your social connectivity, leading to stronger relationships, a more supportive network and a more prosperous, connected life.

Building a meaningful social connection takes time and effort, so be patient and open to new experiences. Developing solid relationships involves mutual trust and respect, so nurturing those connections is the key to maintaining and deepening your social network. Like losing weight or getting fitter, social connection requires consistency, so prioritise it when you least feel like it.

After a few weeks and some meaningful, deep, sometimes frustrating Zoom conversation, Peter and I agreed that he needed to find peers or like-minded people to talk to, socialise with or, more importantly, laugh with. After all, he was not the lone wolf; plenty of expats in Hong Kong have experienced precisely what Peter was feeling.

Nevertheless, like anything, change will only occur when the individual, in this case Peter, acknowledged and owned the problem (lack of social connectivity) and the solution. One of Peter's early wins was joining the Hong Kong Yacht Club. Not only did it provide him with a much-needed outlet for physical activity, but it also allowed him to meet new people and forge new friendships. The camaraderie and support he found at the yacht club helped Peter feel more settled and content in his new life.

I worked and supported Peter for 12 weeks, and these newfound connections created the perfect therapy. Peter's health, wellbeing and zest for life began to improve. He started eating better, exercising regularly and getting the rest he needed after a long day in the office. His mood lifted and he enjoyed life in Hong Kong more than he ever thought possible. Peter could finally see the benefits and positive effects of relocating to Hong Kong on him personally and professionally, enhancing his career trajectory and, more importantly, enriching his life.

Peter's story is a testament to the importance of social connection for our health and wellbeing. By reaching out, building relationships with others and establishing a 'team,' we can all improve our physical and mental health and find greater happiness and fulfilment in our lives.

What, how, when: the core trio for improving social connectivity

1. What:

- Define your social connectivity goals: Identify what you want to achieve in terms of social connectivity. Clarify the specific outcomes you're aiming for to guide your efforts effectively.
- Social connectivity goals: What do you want to improve? This could include expanding your social network, strengthening existing relationships, becoming more active in your community or enhancing your professional connections.

2. How:

- Develop your strategy: Determine how you will achieve your social connectivity goals. This involves creating actionable strategies and incorporating practices to help you connect with others and build relationships.
- Strategies for improvement: How will you enhance your social connectivity?
    - Expand your network: Attend social events, join clubs or groups and participate in community activities to meet new people.
    - Strengthen relationships: Schedule regular catchups with friends and family, offer support and show appreciation.
    - Enhance professional connections: Engage in networking events, follow up with contacts and contribute to industry groups or forums.

3. When:

- Schedule and integrate social activities: Specify when you will implement your strategies and engage in social activities. Consistency and regularity are vital to building and maintaining connections.

- Social activities schedule: When will you act?
    - Daily: Make small, meaningful interactions, such as checking in with a colleague or friend.
    - Weekly: Plan and participate in social or community events, such as family dinners, friend gatherings or networking meetings.
    - Monthly: Attend more noteworthy events or activities, like community festivals, workshops or volunteer opportunities.

Take the first step towards lasting wellbeing: create your personalised social connectivity plan

Building a strong social network is not just about who you know; it is about understanding the depth of social connectivity. Identify the relationships that truly matter and foster interactions that enrich your life and bring long-lasting value.

Start today! Set specific social goals and take steps to reach them, nurturing a support system that will empower and uplift you well into the future. By focusing on social connectivity's what, how and when, you create a structured approach that helps you systematically build and enhance your social network. This formula ensures you work towards your social goals and maintain meaningful connections over time.

WRITE DOWN YOUR PLAN HERE:

What:
_____
_____
_____
_____
_____
_____

How:
_____
_____
_____
_____
_____
_____

When:
_____
_____
_____
_____
_____
_____

CHAPTER 10

Sex: The role of sex in health and relationships

Why sex needs open communication in long-term relationships

Sex is that dirty word that people don't like to discuss, but most of the population has done it at some stage…

Sex needs to be addressed openly, particularly if you are in a long-term relationship, as someone's needs, desires or passion might change over time. The facts speak for themselves that most heterosexual men prioritise erotic connection. In contrast, most heterosexual women are emotional (*Do we share common goals? Do we like to do things together? Is he intelligent? Is he a family man? Is he a 'provider'?*). By the time she has answered these questions, the man had already taken care of himself. True? Selfish? Other…

Sexual intercourse is a fundamental aspect of human life, deeply intertwined with our physical, emotional and mental wellbeing. Beyond its essential role in reproduction, sexual activity has various physical, psychological and relational benefits that significantly impact men's overall health.

The health benefits of sex: more than just pleasure

When looking to achieve optimal health, sex is a crucial component for blokes as it contributes to overall health and vitality in multiple ways, many of which we have discussed in previous chapters. Sex can boost your immune system, promote cardiovascular health and release endorphins, which reduce stress. Additionally, regular sexual activity may improve sleep quality and even foster emotional intimacy, positively impacting mental wellbeing.

The key is finding someone you have a connection with and if you are in a long-term relationship, it all starts with communication and understanding what you are getting into in the first place.

Sure, there is transactional sex, but for those looking for a more intimate connection, communication and a stable relationship are a good starting point. It is worth considering that relationships change, as do their associated needs. It is not always pleasure, passion, emotion, physical release, excitement, enjoyment or a combination of all the above. You can't always have them all.

Having worked with people for over 20 years, I have multiple stories I could share about infidelity and some that should be made into a Netflix documentary. It is worth understanding that the most common reasons marriages fail are the breakdown of trust, a feeling of anger, betrayal, insecurity or a blend of all these factors.

Emotional connection versus casual encounters: Eddie's story

I remember a client of mine, Eddie, who had been happily married, sharing his life with someone he believed to be his soulmate. But after 11 years of marriage, cracks appeared in their foundation; sex had been a challenge throughout and indeed, towards the end, it was close to non-existent. Eventually, their love crumbled, leaving Eddie divorced and adrift in a sea of uncertainty. Fortunately, Eddie didn't have kids; he married when he was 26 years old, yet he was lost at 37.

At first, Eddie tried to drown his sorrows in the arms of random women, seeking solace in their physical embrace. But no matter how many fleeting encounters he had; he could not shake the feeling of emptiness that consumed him. Each encounter left him feeling hollow as if he was searching for something he couldn't quite name.

Not only was his emotional health at risk, but his physical health was also being jeopardised as he would take part in social activities that didn't complement a balanced lifestyle. This involved poor nutritional habits, inactivity and poor sleep hygiene. Eddie would come to training frustrated, looking for something he couldn't find.

Sure, the frequency of sex wasn't a problem, but the act was leaving him emotionally exhausted. Dating, transacting and then doing it all over again.

Eddie was trapped in a cycle of meaningless flings as the years passed, each further distancing him from the emotional connection he craved. Deep down, he knew something was missing, but he couldn't entirely focus on what it was. It wasn't until he met Sarah that things began to change.

Sarah was different from the other women Eddie had encountered. They were introduced through friends and the beginning of their relationship was very platonic. Many months into the friendship, he thought it could become a relationship; the warmth in her eyes and her smile drew him in, sparking a glimmer of hope in his heart. Every week, I would get an update on his progress and I knew he had strong feelings toward Sarah, but he was in the denial stage, trying to protect himself emotionally.

The relationship didn't get off to the perfect start. Eddie was guarded, hesitant to open up after being hurt so many times before when he was busy looking.

Fortunately, Sarah was patient and understanding of the walls he had built around himself. She encouraged him to be vulnerable and share his fears and insecurities to avoid fear of judgment.

Eddie slowly but surely began to let down his defences, allowing Sarah to see the real him beneath the facade he had constructed. Eddie opened up as their relationship continued to prosper and he found that Sarah did the same, sharing her hopes, dreams, fears and doubts.

As time passed, the bond grew through their connection. The critical ingredient of their relationship was honesty, vulnerability and open communication, qualities Eddie had never truly experienced when using dating apps. As they navigated the ups and downs of life together, Eddie realised that this was what he had been searching for all along. The difference was the strong connection emotionally and mentally, which just enhanced the physical attraction and joy they both experienced sexually. I remember him telling me that when they started having sex, it was so different, so much better and so much more fulfilling than any casual sexual experience.

Building strong relationships: the role of honesty and vulnerability

Like all relationships, it was challenging. There were arguments and misunderstandings, moments of doubt and uncertainty. But through it all, Eddie and Sarah stood by each other, facing whatever challenges came their way with unwavering support and love.

Eddie learned that relationships weren't always easy, but the rewards were worth the effort. Through honesty, vulnerability and open communication, he had found the emotional connection he had been missing for so long. He would verbalise that when he looked into Sarah's eyes, he knew he had finally found his soulmate, someone he could share his life with in all its beautiful imperfections.

Too many of us give up when the going gets tough, but as I always preach, 'run your body like a business,' and your relationship should be no different. Expect there to be tough times, frustrating times and times when you wonder *why?*. The upside of a loving, sharing and caring relationship is so much more significant than transactional sex that has little emotional connection. So, my advice, if you are in a relationship is to stay physically and emotionally connected.

The impact of equality on sexual satisfaction in relationships

Having personally been off the 'transactional' sex circuit for well over two decades, I think it is essential to recognise that as relationships grow and develop, so does one's sex life, and at times, this might directly impact the quality and frequency of your sex life. There are obvious reasons for this, like starting a family, having kids and work commitments. During my research, I came across a study called 'Egalitarianism, Housework and Sexual Frequency in Marriage,' which appeared in the *American Sociological Review* (Kornrich et al 2013). This study went against the logic but certainly supported my theory that as the marriage improves by becoming more equal, the sex in the marriage will improve too. The study found that when men did not do certain chores around the house, couples had less sex. Tools down, I hear you shout!

As the world progresses and equal opportunities evolve to level out the domestic playing field, what impact has this had on your relationship? In the next chapter on bio-individuality, I discuss that what is right for one person isn't necessarily suitable for another as everyone's relationships, expectations and environments differ. Many factors need to be considered when looking at ways to strengthen one's relationship and sex is only one component of a flourishing relationship.

Over the years, I have certainly changed my thinking around the roles and responsibilities within the family environment and I am now an advocate for progressive marriages. Hence, you support each other's careers, passions and hobbies, but the outcome must be a family/relationship-orientated end goal, inside and outside the bedroom. Communication and clarity around your sexual desire and preferences are the foundation for a fruitful sex life, but it does take two to tango. So, speak your thoughts before diving into your actions.

Sexual activity, like any physical exertion, increases heart rate and circulation. It also triggers the release of endorphins, which means it can lower stress and anxiety levels. There have also been studies that support that regular sex can boost your immune system (Lorenz 2014). A satisfying sex life can also contribute to a positive self-image and personal self-esteem.

I am not a sex therapist, but I think it is essential to establish some boundaries when considering the relationship blueprint that you both agree on. Remember, we all have needs, wants and desires; some are quite different, but you must be open and honest. An excellent place to start is by creating bedroom boundaries and expectations. Don't reflect on your past; that will only fuel your ego, not your urges. Just ask Eddie.

Finally, when it comes to sexual wellbeing and relationships, it is essential to respect and understand that it is deeply personal and there is no one-size (pardon the pun) solution. Nevertheless, not all blokes crave sex all the time, just the majority.

Andropause

The topic of menopause or perimenopause often overshadows the male equivalent of andropause, which can have a significant impact on one's sex life. Analogous to menopause, andropause is a condition characterised by a gradual decline in testosterone levels and other hormonal changes that can affect men's health and quality of life.

Typically, when your testosterone test result are low, your sex drive is also low. This is why I encourage all of my male clientele to get regular blood profiling so I can look at specific blood markers, particularly testosterone, which gradually declines during andropause and significantly impacts one's health.

As I mentioned in Chapter 6, lower testosterone levels have been linked to an increased risk of cardiovascular disease. Another side effect of andropause is that it can lead to metabolic syndrome, which is characterised by high blood pressure, high blood sugar, excess body fat around the waist and abnormal cholesterol levels. These symptoms increase the risk of diabetes and heart disease.

As you get older, your bone density also decreases, which usually correlates with a decrease in testosterone. For some men, the psychological impact of andropause can lead to depression, anxiety and a diminished sense of wellbeing. Although andropause is a natural part of ageing and the signs and symptoms aren't as drastic as menopause, it is essential to manage it and the most effective way to do this is through the fundamentals: nutrition, exercise and sleep.

Maintaining a balanced nutritional plan that includes adequate protein sources, fruit, vegetables, and foods that boost testosterone levels, such as zinc and Vitamin D, will undoubtedly be a proactive approach. Regular exercise, both aerobic (Zone 2) and strength training, is imperative as we age, and this will certainly minimise the effects of andropause, along with adequate sleep.

Although andropause is often dismissed, or for many people there is a real lack of awareness/education around it, it is still a significant phase in a man's life. I believe there needs to be greater awareness, education and support for blokes as we age, hence my passion for writing this book and creating the Blokes Inc. community. Together, we need to improve awareness and build a proactive movement to minimise the effects ageing has on men's health. Perhaps I have got a little sidetracked, but if you want to improve your sex life there needs to be a proactive movement to minimise the effects of ageing.

The key to an improved sex life is to prioritise communication, emotional connection and mutual respect to enhance sexual intimacy and compatibility. These are the key ingredients (foreplay if you like). By following this blueprint, you can hopefully work towards optimising your wellbeing in your sexual and romantic relationships.

The hidden struggles of sexual addiction

For me, sex is a natural and healthy aspect of human life and something that you should respect and maintain regardless of your age. Still, when it becomes an uncontrollable obsession, it can lead to sex addiction. Like any addiction, sex addiction can have severe consequences on an individual's mental, emotional and relational wellbeing. Sex addiction is a complex and challenging issue that can significantly compromise an individual's wellbeing. It becomes an obsession, hence the saying 'one-track mind.'

For many sex addicts, it is their constant thoughts and desires that lead to anxiety, depression and other emotional disorders, further exacerbating existing mental health issues. The constant need for sexual fulfilment can result in emotional turmoil. Feelings of guilt and shame are common among individuals grappling with sex addiction. It is this emotional strain that can contribute to a cycle of compulsive behaviour as people with addiction seek temporary relief through further sexual encounters.

For those individuals in 'transitional' or open relationships, sex addiction can take a toll on physical health. Addicts tend to engage in risky behaviours, exposing themselves to sexually transmitted infections. Not dissimilar to other physical endeavours, the relentless pursuit of sexual gratification may lead to exhaustion, sleep deprivation and neglect of other essential aspects of self-care, as addicts are so one-dimensional.

Unfortunately, sex addiction can strain and destroy relationships. The secrecy and deception often associated with this condition can erode trust between partners. Typically, under these circumstances, intimacy may suffer as the addicted individual may prioritise their compulsions over the emotional connection. Similar to a gambling addiction, the pursuit of sexual gratification may come at a considerable financial cost. Individuals with sex addiction may spend exorbitant amounts of money on pornography, escorts or other sexual activities.

Porn addiction

Similar to sex addiction, porn addiction can also have detrimental effects on men's health, both physically and mentally. One significant impact that tends to be an afterthought is the potential for erectile dysfunction. Excessive consumption of pornography may desensitise individuals, leading to difficulties in achieving and maintaining erections during real-life sexual encounters. This can create performance anxiety and further strain relationships.

Porn addiction may also contribute to a distorted perception of intimacy and body image. Men exposed to unrealistic depictions of sex may develop unrealistic expectations, causing dissatisfaction in their relationships. This can lead to a cycle of discontent, further fuelling the reliance on pornography as an escape from real-life complexities. The same scenario as sex addicts is also evident in those that seek porn. Their mental health is at risk, as porn addiction often leads to increased feelings of guilt, shame and isolation.

Men struggling with either sex or porn addiction may experience a decline in self-esteem and self-worth, negatively affecting their overall mental wellbeing. Additionally, excessive engagement in either sex or porn can disrupt your normal dopamine regulation in the brain, similar to other addictive behaviours, which then results in a decreased ability to experience pleasure in everyday activities, potentially leading to depression.

Like all other addictions, addressing the adverse effects of porn addiction requires a multifaceted approach. This can start by simply promoting sexual education that includes discussions about healthy relationships, consent and the difficult topics of casual sex or porn.

For me, sex is like a packet of party mix. It is always good; you occasionally crave it more than others and it is hard to stop once you start. There is a sudden high before adrenal exhaustion, and if you *choose*, you can share it with others.

Six-step blueprint to help you in the bedroom

Step 1: Open and honest communication

Start by having open and honest conversations with your partner about desires, needs and boundaries. It is so challenging yet essential, particularly in heterosexual relationships, as needs and desires change as genders age. The key is to start by creating a safe space for discussing your sexual preferences and concerns.

Listen actively and empathetically to your partner's perspective and try to understand their needs.

Step 2. Build emotional connection

Work on strengthening the emotional connection with your partner. Engage in activities that promote intimacy, such as spending quality time together, expressing appreciation and showing affection.

Explore ways to bond emotionally, as a deeper emotional connection often leads to improved sexual intimacy and compatibility.

Step 3: Explore and experience

Be open to trying new things in the bedroom, experimenting with different sexual activities and discovering what both you and your partner(s) enjoy. Prioritise consent, respect and mutual pleasure in any sexual exploration.

Step 4: Prioritise self-care and wellbeing

Focus on your own physical and mental wellbeing, as this can have a positive impact on your sexual health and satisfaction.

Get regular exercise, eat a balanced diet, manage stress and get enough sleep to promote overall vitality.

Step 5: Seek professional guidance

If you are facing difficulties that are impacting your sexual intimacy and relationship, don't hesitate to seek the guidance of a qualified therapist who specialises in sexual health and relationships.

Step 6: Build a framework

Consider what you and your better half want and build a framework that suits your appetite.

Some aspects of your framework might be:

- to share or not share the 'party mix'
- design versus desire
- open communication
- safe practices
- emotional connection
- frequency.

What, how, when: The core trio for improving your sex life

1. What:

- Define your sex life goals: Identify what aspects of your sex life you want to improve or enhance. Clear goals will help you focus your efforts and measure progress.
- Sex life goals: What specific areas do you want to address? This could include improving intimacy, increasing frequency, exploring new experiences, enhancing communication with your partner or addressing any issues related to sexual health.

2. How:

- Develop a plan for enhancement: Determine how you will achieve your goals for improving your sex life. This involves creating actionable strategies and incorporating practices that support your objectives.
- Strategies for improvement: How will you enhance your sex life?
    - Communication: Discuss your desires, preferences and concerns with your partner. Effective communication fosters intimacy and understanding.
    - Exploration: Try new experiences or activities, such as new techniques, settings or routines, that you and your partner are comfortable with.
    - Education: Educate yourself and your partner about sexual health and wellness. Consider reading books, attending workshops or seeking professional advice if needed.
    - Emotional connection: Strengthen your emotional bond with your partner through shared activities, quality time and mutual support.

3. When:

- Schedule and integrate enhancements: Specify when you will implement your strategies and practices. Consistency and intention are vital to making improvements in your sex life.
- Enhancement schedule: When will you focus on these aspects?
    - Daily: Engage in small actions that build intimacy, such as affectionate gestures, meaningful conversations and quality time together.
    - Weekly: Plan activities or date nights that foster connection and exploration. Schedule time for discussions about your sex life and desires.
    - Monthly: Assess your progress and adjust as needed. Set aside time for more in-depth discussions, try new activities or seek professional guidance if necessary.

Take the first step towards lasting wellbeing: create your personalised intimacy plan

By taking a strategic approach to improving your sex life—focusing on the what, how and when—you not only build a framework for lasting change, but also create opportunities for deeper connection and greater satisfaction. This approach allows you to address your individual needs, communicate openly with your partner and overcome the challenges that may arise in a relationship. Start by prioritising intimacy, setting goals and having open conversations about your desires and boundaries. Remember, improving your sex life is a journey, not a one-time fix, and it is something you can continually work on together. Take action now—be proactive, explore new ways to connect and invest in a healthier, more fulfilling sexual relationship.

WRITE DOWN YOUR PLAN HERE:

What:

_____
_____
_____
_____
_____
_____

How:

_____
_____
_____
_____
_____
_____

When:

_____
_____
_____
_____
_____
_____

CHAPTER 11

Bio-individuality: one size does not fit all

Be yourself; everyone else is already taken.

—Oscar Wilde

Creating your healthier self

Having surpassed well over 20,000 individual training sessions, I have enough personal, emotional, physical, psychological and physiological knowledge to discuss bio-individuality and why it is essential for your long-term wellness success.

I am continually frustrated that we have more access to information and education, yet all health-related biometrics globally are worsening. You only need to look at the prevalence of obesity, the number of people who are suffering from Type 2 diabetes and the rise of hypertension and high cholesterol in the community. Not to mention the increased number of people with depression and/or anxiety and the impact that it is having not only on individuals but the broader community.

If nothing else, I am a realist. Many of you reading this book may already have one or more of these 'lifestyle' diseases, frustrated that you haven't got the results you were after having previously attempted a health intervention. I have seen this time and time again. 'My friend did this.' 'I saw this on Instagram.' 'A friend of a friend does this'…but just because it worked for them doesn't necessarily mean it will work for you.

More often than not, the initial action is instigated by an emotional choice, hoping that things will change, rather than seeking help from a paid professional to make educated choices, typically backed by science specific to your needs, goals and health history. So, as you read *Blokes Inc. Play a Bigger Game*, now is the time to reflect on what you have learnt and audit your lifestyle to become multidimensional. Think about your pain points that you would like to improve and commit to taking action to create a better version of *you*.

Understanding why a one-size-fits-all approach does not work for wellness

In this chapter, I will discuss my own experiences around bio-individuality. I'll be the first to admit my diet isn't perfect. I don't count calories; I eat the occasional fast-food meal and enjoy a glass of red wine and a beer with my mates. I don't exercise every day but everything I do is consistent. I prioritise a sleep routine and daily supplementation and focus on having 150 mL of water every waking hour. I encourage you to reflect on your lifestyle and commit to creating change that will lead to a healthier, but more importantly happier version of you, version 2.0.

But remember, a healthy, happy, and functional lifestyle requires combined effort, honesty, intention, and implementation. So, to help you become multidimensional, let's start with your lifestyle audit.

Complete the following lifestyle audit by reflecting on how you manage each of these elements in your life.

Designing your own health audit

Creating a personalised health audit is a powerful step toward taking control of your wellbeing. It begins with a thorough lifestyle review, examining key areas influencing your health and happiness. These include:

- **Sleep:** Assess the quality and duration of your sleep. Are you consistently getting restorative rest?

- **Nutrition:** Review your dietary habits. Are you fuelling your body with nutrient-dense, balanced meals?

- **Exercise:** Consider your physical activity levels. Are you engaging in regular exercise that supports your fitness goals?

- **Stress:** Evaluate your stress levels and coping mechanisms. Is stress a daily struggle, and how are you managing it?

- **Social connectivity:** Reflect on your relationships. Are you maintaining meaningful connections with family, friends and your community?

- **Finance:** Look at your financial health. Are money concerns adding to your stress or limiting your lifestyle choices?

- **Purpose:** Examine your sense of purpose. Do you feel aligned with your life's goals and values?

Identifying pain points

Once you have completed your review, it is time to pinpoint the areas that need the most attention. There are typically two to four pain points as they rarely present in isolation. These pain points might be:

- **Stress:** Chronic stress was affecting my physical and mental health.

- **Relationship/Marriage:** Communication breakdowns and a lack of connection strained my marriage.

- **Weight gain and lack of fitness:** I noticed a gradual decline in my fitness levels and an increase in weight, impacting my energy and confidence.

- **Depression:** The combination of these factors was contributing to feelings of hopelessness and low motivation.

Prioritising and action planning

After identifying your pain points, try prioritising them based on their impact and urgency. In the above example, this may be stress, as it was exacerbating all other issues. Then, once you have addressed stress, you might look into relationship challenges, understanding that a strong, supportive partnership is crucial for overall wellbeing. This would then lead to weight management and fitness, as improving these would boost your physical and mental health. Finally, you might tackle the underlying depression, ensuring you have the tools and support to stay mentally resilient. If you decide you do not, then seek professional advice/assistance.

Call to action

With priorities set, then develop a clear action plan:

- **Stress management:** To reduce work-related stress, implement daily mindfulness practices, such as meditation and breathing exercises, and set firm boundaries.

- **Relationship building:** Schedule weekly check-ins with your partner, focusing on open communication and quality time together.

- **Fitness and nutrition:** Commit to a structured exercise routine and a balanced meal plan that supports weight loss and energy levels.

- **Mental health support:** Seek therapy or coaching to address depression and build coping strategies.

The key to success lies in consistency, structure and accountability. Whether through a coach, a support group or a trusted friend, having someone keep you on track makes all the difference. Now, it is time to take that first step and commit to your health audit journey.

So, what is bio-individuality?

As the name suggests, bio-individuality refers to the concept that each person has unique nutritional, physical, emotional, psychological and lifestyle needs based on their personalised physiological blueprint, which includes genetics, metabolism, and their individual 'end goal.'

Bio-individuality recognises that what works well for one person (nutrition, exercise, stress management) may not necessarily work the same for another person. In recent years, we have seen social media's impact on an individual's 'emotional' purchases as they become more prevalent in search of dopamine validation.

Most of us are guilty of making some emotional purchase. That powder, that pill, that program, that nutritional plan, on social media because you had 'body envy' and then wonder why it didn't work. Or you aspire to feel like they do, look like they look and are willing to do what others do.

Nevertheless, within a few weeks, you are disheartened because you don't get the results you are after. Why? Because the key ingredient is that all programs need to be personalised. Everything you commit to must suit and be designed for you, including your goals, strengths and weaknesses. For the program to be personalised, many factors must be considered, including your age, gender, genetic variations, metabolic differences, gut microbiome, food sensitivity (don't get me started on this), lifestyle factors and even the environment you live in.

There are many variables for consideration, but the key is to create a sustainable lifestyle blueprint that addresses the fundamentals of nutrition, exercise and sleep at the bare minimum and finally, the critical ingredient, consistency. You will find that changing habits is hard at first and that is why many people fail. Once you commit to the journey, the middle will be messy. Sometimes, you will want to quit and revert to your old habits/lifestyle, but if you stay consistent, the reward will be worth it.

The health and fitness industry is built on the fly-by-nighters, fads and fakes, and as a society, we are all suckers for the quick fix. Sure, generic advice, Dr Google and the standard, one-size-fits-all approach have some merit. It gets you thinking about change.

Yet, tailored health programs that meet your goals are essential to creating long-lasting lifestyle changes and results. The cookie-cutter approach is merely a quick, short-term cash grab. Remember, very few people go to bed broke and wake up a millionaire. Your body is the same; you can't go to sleep obese and wake up buffed.

Considering your distinct physiological characteristics, lifestyle and goals, you must understand your bio-individuality and uniqueness. The only way to do this is to create a personalised lifestyle blueprint that acknowledges these differences. It considers the impact nutrition, physical activity and stress management have on overall health optimisation. Your personalised lifestyle blueprint must consider your age, gender, body type and your medical history, your family's medical history, as well as your nutritional and fitness likes and dislikes. The goal is to create a lifestyle blueprint that is both palatable and, more importantly, sustainable.

It's not about education; it's about implementation

Remember, I constantly encourage bio-individuality because it challenges the one-size-fits-all approach to health optimisation. It enables individuals to take a more personalised and holistic view of their wellbeing. So, as you conclude this book, refresh, review and then restructure your environment to suit your needs, goals and desires. Re-visit each chapter and look at your core trio for each topic: your what, your how and your when.

Identify what dimension is having the most significant negative impacts on your health at this point. Is it your current stress levels that are affecting your sleep habits? Or your lack of energy levels causing your emotional eating issues, which has increased your alcohol intake, giving you no desire to exercise?

It is essential to acknowledge that most of you will require different strategies to achieve and maintain good health. For example, some of you may thrive on a high-protein diet, while others may do better with a more plant-based approach.

Similarly, some of you may benefit from high-intensity exercise, while others prefer a more moderate and sustainable routine. This is when I encourage you to take ownership of your program, lifestyle and the associated outcomes. Don't let emotions dictate your end goals. You are an educated human being. You are reading this book because you want to create change; now, the only way to do this is to be honest and upfront with yourself.

Throughout this book, we covered many topics when looking at ways we could create change to optimise your health and wellbeing. At the start of *Blokes Inc. Play a Bigger Game*, we went deep into mindfulness, motivation and habits, and we established that you must control all three to create change. When it comes to mindfulness, you name it, I have tried it, but the only modality that fills my cup or slows down my grey matter, giving me clarity, is long-distance running.

When I run, my mind slows, the white noise dissipates, I relax, my breathing rate becomes consistent and my cortisol levels lower. I have tried yoga, meditation, breath work, visualisation, journalling and numerous sensory exercises, but nothing has the same effect as running. Many people find meditation beneficial, while others may prefer mindful movement practices like yoga or tai chi. It doesn't matter what it is; what matters is that you find what resonates with you to cultivate a sense of presence and awareness.

Reflect on your mindfulness practice if you have one or have tried one, what works for you? The key is to identify how you felt before and afterwards. You may need to try a few different modalities until you find one that works but make a start.

Assess your number one dimension for change

When analysing your health audit, what is the top area that needs attention? After reviewing clients' health audits over many years, I've found that nutrition is the most common area people struggle with in their personalised lifestyle plans.

If you break it down to its simplest form, it returns to the fundamentals. Try to modify your eating habits around seasonal eating, control your portion sizes, include plenty of colours (fruit and vegetables), ensure you consume good protein sources with every meal, minimise your packaged/processed food intake and cut down or eliminate your refined sugars.

I discussed nutrition in Chapters 3 and 4; for most people, it is the most problematic dimension to get right. Why? More often than not, people's stress response is brought upon by 'emotion,' leading to poor nutritional choices. Think about it—you have a stressful day; you might find alcohol is the answer. You fight with your spouse, partner, friend or family member and then you binge eat. You are tired, so you have a hit of sugar, chocolate or caffeine for that immediate pick-me-up to keep you going. Typically, I am great between breakfast and dinner and a little more relaxed when eating with the family.

Nevertheless, I still ensure I hit my protein intake (2 g/kg body weight), take my supplements and drink plenty of water. I minimise packaged produce and consume many colours of fruits and vegetables. My ideal advice is to experiment with what works for you and your lifestyle (work, friends, family commitments) and find a nutritional approach that works best for your body and mind. It just needs to be easy to be sustainable.

Whatever it is, bio-individuality needs to form the framework. In Chapters 5 and 6, we went deep into exercise; the type, intensity, duration and frequency will dictate the results. Some of you might love exercise, and it's part of your DNA, but exercise is a chore for most of you.

Remember, though, that whatever you do, my formula is to be better than average, so use this as your guide for implementing exercise in your blueprint. There are 52 weeks a year, so to be better than average include 'structured' exercise for 45 weeks out of those 52 weeks. There are 60 minutes in an hour, so any exercise over 30 minutes is better than average, but I'd go as far as to say that something is better than nothing if your baseline is zero.

I went through a stage where I loved lifting heavy weights and I did this for years; then, I got into ultra-marathon running and ran 14 ultra-marathons ranging from 50–100 km, including 12 marathons. Now I'm older and wiser, I enjoy a blend of weights, water sports and a little bit of running.

The key is to find an exercise routine that is enjoyable and sustainable for you. Nevertheless, when it comes to resistance training, I firmly believe that everyone should lift weights at least three times per week, regardless of age and gender. There is enough scientific evidence to support this. Many of you may think resistance training is boring, but the benefits will outweigh any negative feelings.

Stress is another dirty word that affects us all differently, yet it is essential to remember that not all stress is bad. Reflect on stressful situations that trigger your pain points, acute or chronic. How could you deal with these stressors differently?

Remember, depending on what type of stress you are under, your body responds differently. In certain stressful situations, you might eat poorly, drink alcohol more frequently, exercise less, experience disrupted sleeping patterns, minimise social connectivity and remove yourself from friends and family. Therefore, it is imperative to understand your unique stress response and develop a personalised stress management technique that lowers your cortisol and balances your mind and body.

This personalised stress management technique could include breathwork, music, meditation, sunlight, comedy, et cetera. For me, it's getting out in nature, running, jumping in the water or going to the gym. The key to stress reduction is changing the environment, which will change your state. If my environment doesn't allow this, my backup plan is to listen to music to change my thoughts. The key is to do something that changes your current state of play (mind), which will then positively impact your physiology.

Much of my passion is helping humans optimise their performance and, for many, their quality of life. I aspire to help people live a happier, healthier, more fulfilling life they are passionate about. So, when it comes to longevity, social connection is crucial. Maintaining strong connections with friends, family and the community has been linked to numerous benefits, including reduced stress, increased sense of belonging and improved mental health. People with close relationships tend to be happier, more confident and better able to cope with life's challenges.

Earlier in the book, I spoke about creating your team and having a supportive network that complements your passion, purpose and potential. The best businesses, sporting teams and organisations all have an effective team behind them. Studies have shown that people with strong social connections tend to live longer, healthier lives (Holt-Lunstad 2015). They are less likely to experience chronic diseases such as heart disease and depression and they are more likely to engage in healthy behaviours.

Social connectivity can also help reduce feelings of loneliness and isolation, known risk factors for poor health outcomes. An excellent example of this was my client, Peter, who moved from Melbourne to Hong Kong. He knew something was wrong, but he didn't realise that his lack of social connection and social isolation were impacting his health, both physically and emotionally.

Many of you have heard about the 'blue zones,' which refer to regions worldwide where people live much longer than average. These areas, which include places like Okinawa, Japan and Ikaria, Greece, have populations with elevated levels of social connectivity. In these communities, people often live in close-knit, supportive environments where they interact regularly with others. This social interaction provides emotional support and encourages healthy behaviours such as regular physical activity, healthy eating and a sense of purpose. Therefore, connecting with friends, family and the community is essential for happiness and health. Solid social connections can improve an individual's quality of life and longevity.

When it comes to sex, I wish I was the expert and if you speak to the majority of blokes, we always want more. Yet it is not always about the quantity, as Eddie mentioned in Chapter 10. Sex is a complex and multifaceted aspect of human life, influenced by biological, psychological and social factors. When it comes to bio-individuality, it is crucial to recognise that each person is unique and this uniqueness extends to their sexuality. Understanding and embracing this concept is essential for promoting healthy attitudes and behaviours related to sex.

One of the critical aspects of bio-individuality concerning sex is that what works for one person may not work for another. This applies to sexual orientations, desires and responses. In this day and age, embracing bio-individuality in sex also means acknowledging the diversity of sexual orientations and identities. Each person's experience of their sexuality is valid and deserving of respect.

I recommend talking openly about your desires, preferences, and concerns. There are many dynamics to consider for both partners, and open communication can help each person understand the other's needs. With this understanding, you can work together to keep the sexual aspect of your relationship fulfilling, even as you face challenges like children, stress, menopause, andropause, or ageing.

Unfortunately, the desire ebbs and flows for some, but this doesn't mean the relationship is unhealthy or the desire is gone forever. Sometimes, stress, fatigue or other life challenges can temporarily dampen one's passion. By staying connected, being open and working together, couples can navigate these changes and keep their relationship strong and fulfilling. But like anything you do, being open and honest is essential. Communication and clarity around your sexual desire and preferences are the foundation for a fruitful sex life.

Consider your unique needs and circumstances when embracing bio-individuality concerning men's health and taking a personalised approach to wellness. If all men took this proactive approach, 'lifestyle' diseases would decrease dramatically, science and knowledge would overpower one's emotions and men would all be happier and, more importantly, healthier. Blokes are constantly told that we aren't 'emotional' enough, so let this be the ignitor of your emotional wellbeing and design a personalised blueprint that suits you.

When designing your personalised blueprint, consider addressing the following five steps, many of which you have addressed in earlier chapters.

Five-step blueprint for improving bio-individuality

1. Assess your personal needs and baselines

Begin by understanding your unique biological and psychological characteristics. Conduct a comprehensive assessment to establish your baselines in critical areas such as mindset, exercise, nutrition, sleep, stress, social connectivity and sex.

Use tools like health assessments, genetic testing, personal health data and psychological evaluations. This assessment helps identify your specific needs, preferences and areas for improvement.

2. Set personalised goals and priorities

Set goals and priorities that reflect your individual needs. Build self-awareness, mental resilience, and set personal objectives across various areas: develop a fitness routine suited to your body and preferences, create a diet plan that fits your nutritional needs and tastes, establish healthy sleep habits, apply stress management techniques tailored to your triggers, and nurture meaningful relationships that support your social preferences. Address aspects of sexual health and intimacy that align with your personal and relational values.

3. Develop a customised action plan

Create an action plan tailored to your goals, including specific practices that align with your needs. For mindset, engage in activities like journalling or therapy to build resilience. Develop a workout routine suited to your fitness level, interests, and resources. Plan meals that meet your dietary needs and lifestyle. Create a bedtime routine that supports restful sleep and choose stress-reducing activities that help you manage stress effectively. Build a social calendar that aligns with your relationship goals and communicate your needs for greater satisfaction and intimacy in personal relationships.

4. Monitor and adjust your plan regularly

Continuously track your progress in each area and adjust as needed. Regularly review how well your strategies work and align with your bio-individual needs.

- Progress tracking: Use tools like health apps, journals or regular check-ins to monitor your progress.
- Adjustments: Based on feedback and outcomes, tweak your strategies and goals to better suit your evolving needs and circumstances.

5. Seek support and professional guidance

Engage with professionals and support networks to enhance your journey towards improved bio-individuality. This may include consulting with healthcare providers, nutritionists, personal trainers, mental health professionals or relationship counsellors.

- Professional guidance: Seek expert advice tailored to your unique needs for personalised recommendations and support.
- Support networks: Connect with communities or groups with similar health goals and interests to gain motivation and share experiences.

This blueprint will create a comprehensive, personalised approach to improving bio-individuality across various aspects of your life, leading to a more balanced and fulfilling lifestyle.

By embracing bio-individuality, you can take control of your wellbeing, make informed choices and support your unique health needs. Over the years in the wellness industry, I have found that this approach promotes better health outcomes and empowers blokes to participate actively in their health and wellness journey.

I have worked with thousands of people, so I know that everyone has different pain points and coping mechanisms for dealing with stress. Some find solace in meditation, while others prefer exercising or engaging in other creative activities. Others might try all these options and see a health professional to give them tools, guidance, advice, support and expertise. The key is to identify which chosen support mechanism aligns with your needs at the time under your current environment.

Embrace bio-individuality and unlock the limitless possibilities in pursuing optimal health and fitness. Stop following social media handles, your mates' programs or routines, and stop being brainwashed by influencers who might be aesthetically fit but physiologically and psychologically unfit. Design and implement a blueprint that suits *you*.

It is essential to understand that promoting bio-individuality is not just a practice; it is a philosophy that fosters wellbeing, enhances self-awareness and empowers you to take charge in your unique way.

So, ask yourself:

- What is *your* optimal health?

- What do *you* need to change?

- What are *you* willing to sacrifice?

- What does *your* lifestyle blueprint look like?

What, how, when: the core trio for bio-individuality

1. What:

- Define your bio-individuality goals: Identify what specific aspects of your bio-individuality you want to address or improve. This involves understanding your unique needs and setting clear, tailored objectives.

- Bio-individuality goals: What areas do you want to focus on? This could include optimising your mindset, exercise, nutrition, sleep, stress management, social connectivity and sex according to your needs and preferences.

2. How:

- Develop a personalised strategy: Determine how you will achieve your bio-individuality goals. Create a plan with specific actions and practices tailored to your unique characteristics.

- Personalised strategy: How will you implement changes?
    - Mindset: Incorporate practices like mindfulness, cognitive-behavioural techniques or personal development exercises that suit your mental health needs.
    - Exercise: Develop a fitness plan that fits your physical condition and preferences, such as strength training, cardio or flexibility exercises.
    - Nutrition: Create a diet plan based on your metabolic needs, food sensitivities and taste preferences. Include meal planning and nutritional tracking.
    - Sleep: Establish a sleep routine and environment tailored to your sleep patterns and requirements.
    - Stress management: Use stress reduction techniques that align with your stress triggers and coping style, such as relaxation exercises, hobbies or time management strategies.

- Social connectivity: Engage in social activities and build relationships that match your social preferences and goals.
- Sex: Explore and communicate your needs and preferences to improve intimacy and sexual satisfaction.

3. When:

- Schedule and implement your plan: Specify when you will implement your personalised strategies. Consistency and timing are vital to making effective changes.
- Implementation schedule: When will you act?
    - Daily: Integrate small, consistent actions into your daily routine, such as mindfulness practices, meal planning or short exercise sessions.
    - Weekly: Plan and review your weekly activities, including workouts, social interactions and stress management practices.
    - Monthly: Assess your progress, adjust your strategies if needed and set aside time for comprehensive reviews of your bio-individuality goals.

Take the first step towards lasting wellbeing: create your bio-individuality plan

By focusing on bio-individuality's what, how and when, you set the foundation for a highly personalised and well-structured approach to optimising your health and wellbeing. Understanding that no two people are the same is critical—what works for one person might not work for another. By tailoring your strategies to fit your unique needs, preferences and biological makeup, you create a health plan that works with your body, not against it. This approach helps you make informed decisions about your diet, exercise, sleep and stress management, ensuring that every action you take is purposeful and effective.

Consistency is crucial in this process, and by integrating these individualised strategies into your routine, you'll see more sustainable and meaningful results over time. Reassessing and adjusting is important if you are not seeing the progress you expect. Your health blueprint is not static—it should evolve as you learn more about what works for you. Do not be afraid to try new methods, refine your approach and continue adjusting. Act now, reflect on your current approach and commit to making changes to help you become the best version of yourself.

WRITE DOWN YOUR PLAN HERE:

What:

_____
_____
_____
_____
_____
_____

How:

_____
_____
_____
_____
_____
_____

When:

_____
_____
_____
_____
_____
_____

CHAPTER 12

Your legacy

Some people die at age 25 but are not buried until 75.

—Benjamin Franklin

What will you be remembered for?

As you reach the end of your journey with *Blokes Inc. Play a Bigger Game* hopefully, it has become clear that the principles of running your body like a business are not just beneficial but essential for a long, fulfilling life. Health optimisation, honesty, consistency and personal health accountability are the cornerstones of this approach, ensuring that every aspect of your wellbeing is meticulously managed and continuously improved. When this occurs, you are 'multidimensional.'

Just as a successful business continually seeks to optimise its operations, so should you strive to enhance your wellness profile. Health optimisation involves taking a proactive approach to wellbeing, focusing on the factors contributing to one's physical, mental and emotional health. There needs to be structure, standards and non-negotiables, so too respecting that regular exercise is a non-negotiable, creating and maintaining a balanced nutritional plan, as well as ensuring sufficient sleep and having a stress management strategy.

You should also gain a thirst for knowledge and stay informed about the latest health research. At times, you should be open to new methods and practices to improve your overall health, reflecting on bio-individuality. At times, you might feel as though you are failing, not getting the results you are after, but at no stage is failure a bad thing.

Case study: Jake reframes failure

For many, failure is perceived as a setback or a roadblock that hinders progress. However, reframing failure as a positive force can transform your approach to achieving your wellness goals. Embracing failure builds resilience and provides invaluable lessons that propel you toward tremendous success in the future. I remember when I was contracting to a drug and alcohol clinic and a client came in struggling with a deep, dark battle against alcoholism.

After years of destructive behaviour, Jake finally sought help through a six-week treatment program. He poured over $300,000 into his recovery, determined to reclaim his life from the clutches of addiction.

In rehab, Jake made remarkable progress, he adhered to the program diligently, attending therapy sessions, participating in group discussions and embracing a healthier lifestyle. His transformation was evident to everyone around him and by the end of the program, he seemed like a new person.

With a renewed sense of purpose and hope, Jake left the rehab facility, ready to face the world sober. The transition back to everyday life proved more challenging than anticipated. The pressures of work, relationships (single father with four kids) and old environments began to take their toll. The demons he had fought so hard to conquer slowly crept back in.

Despite his best efforts, Jake relapsed. The relapse was not just a slip; it spiralled into a more bottomless abyss than he had ever experienced. Jake found himself in a darker place than before, consumed by guilt, shame and hopelessness. He felt let down and disillusioned with the clinic. He was angry, having invested so much money in the clinic and had little to no contact with the organisation afterwards. Having worked in rehab clinics for over a decade, I have yet to find one that offers ongoing, available and, more importantly, viable home-based treatment options.

It was at this critical juncture that Jake reached out to me. Recognising the severity of his situation, I knew Jake needed a different approach. We began working together, delving deep into his experiences, fears and failures. Instead of focusing solely on the relapse, we reframed his thinking around it. I helped Jake understand that failure was not the end of his journey but an integral part of his path to recovery. We explored the reasons behind his relapse and identified triggers and vulnerabilities.

This introspection was not about assigning blame but gaining insight and learning from the experience. Jake started seeing his relapse not as a defeat but as a valuable lesson. We developed strategies he could implement should he face such triggers in the future, incorporating new coping mechanisms and building a robust support network.

Failure as a tool for growth

By using failure as a tool for growth, Jake learned to adapt and evolve. Failure is a unique learning opportunity that success often does not offer. Failure is a positive when you can find the solution, the formula and the answers. When you fail, you gain insights into what doesn't work, allowing you to refine your strategies and methods.

By analysing Jake's mistakes, we could better understand his needs and responses, creating a more effective and personalised wellness plan moving forward. Through Jake's previous failures and setbacks, he became more self-aware, which allowed him to recognise the early signs of any potential triggers or signs of a relapse. We focused on creating a sustainable lifestyle that prioritised his wellbeing, incorporating regular therapy, exercise and mindfulness practices.

Jake's journey was far from easy, but with perseverance and a shift in perspective, he began to rebuild his life. He understood that setbacks were not indicators of weakness but opportunities for resilience and strength. He understood the importance of creating a team that added value and personal health accountability.

By embracing his failures, Jake became more resilient, adaptive and prepared for future challenges. The key learning is that life is tricky; you will always face challenges and setbacks, but if you follow the process and reflect on your behaviours, you will build character and increase your chances of success.

Today, Jake continues to work on his sobriety with a renewed sense of purpose. He uses his past failures as a stepping stone, learning from each experience and growing stronger with every step. His story is a testament to the power of resilience and the importance of viewing failure as a catalyst for change.

Jake transformed his darkest moments into the foundation for a brighter, healthier future by reframing his thinking and futureproofing his strategies. If, at some point, you find yourself in a comparable situation to Jake, reframe your thinking and take solace in the fact that failure is merely proofing your future.

I see failure as a critical ingredient in your wellness puzzle, along with honesty which is the conjoint of any successful business. Being honest about your habits, challenges and progress will allow you to make informed decisions. It requires acknowledging when you are not meeting your health goals and understanding why. This self-awareness tool will enable you to address any issues head-on rather than ignoring them or making excuses.

Consistency is the key to success

When it comes to success, consistency transforms average businesses into exceptional ones. In the realm of personal health, it's no different. Consistent efforts in maintaining a healthy lifestyle yield significant long-term benefits. Whether it's sticking to a regular workout routine, eating nutritious meals or managing stress effectively, consistency ensures you build and maintain healthy habits that become second nature.

Personal health accountability is about taking responsibility for your health outcomes. It involves setting realistic goals, tracking progress and adjusting as needed. Just as businesses hold regular performance reviews, you should conduct personal health assessments to understand your progress and identify areas for improvement. This accountability will drive you to stay committed to your health goals and strive to improve.

To thrive, a business must diversify and innovate. Similarly, personal health should encompass multiple dimensions—physical, mental, emotional and social wellbeing. Becoming multidimensional means focusing on your physical health and nurturing your mind and relationships. Engaging in activities that stimulate creativity, foster emotional intelligence and build social connections enhances your overall quality of life.

Just as businesses conduct regular audits to ensure they are on track; twice yearly health audits are crucial for personal health optimisation. These audits should involve comprehensive evaluations of your health metrics, such as blood pressure, cholesterol levels, body mass index and mental health assessments. By conducting these audits twice a year, you can identify potential health issues and make any necessary adjustments to your lifestyle.

Twice yearly health audits serve as a reality check, clearly showing your current health status and highlighting areas that need attention. They provide an opportunity to celebrate progress, address shortcomings and renew your commitment to health optimisation.

The legacy...

As *Blokes Inc. Play a Bigger Game* comes to the last chapter, reflect and ask yourself, what legacy would you like to leave? My legacy will be my dedication to men's health, where my passion is educating, inspiring and motivating blokes to take action and become 'multi-dimensional.' I am passionate about optimising personal performance and promoting wellness, but also for building the Blokes Inc. community. In this space, men can thrive, connect and support each other in their journeys.

Beyond my professional impact, a significant driver is my family. My legacy will also reflect the loving and fun family environment Fi and I have cultivated in a cluttered and selfish world. Our legacy will be rich with shared experiences and adventures from around the world, and my life's work will be a testament to the power of connection, care, and living life to its fullest potential.

As you reflect, trust the process and understand that running your body like a business is about achieving health goals and adopting a mindset that prioritises wellbeing in every aspect of life. It's about understanding that your health is your most valuable asset and that investing in it yields the most significant returns. By embracing health optimisation, honesty, consistency, personal health accountability and the art of becoming multidimensional, you can create a legacy of wellness that inspires others to follow suit.

As we close this chapter on *Blokes Inc. Play a Bigger Game*, let's carry forward the lessons learned and continue refining our approach to health.

Commit to:

- regular health audits
- staying honest with yourself
- remaining consistent in your efforts
- embracing a multidimensional approach to wellbeing.

Doing so will improve your health profile and also inspire others to lead healthier, more fulfilling lives.

What, how, when: the core trio for creating a legacy

1. What:

- Define your legacy and life goals: Identify what you want to achieve in creating a meaningful legacy and living a healthier, happier life. Clarify your long-term vision and specific objectives.
- Legacy goals: What impact do you want to make? Consider what you want to be remembered for, such as contributions to your community, advancements in your field, or positive influence on family and friends.
- Health and happiness goals: What improvements do you want to make in your health and happiness? This could include achieving physical fitness, maintaining mental wellbeing, nurturing relationships or pursuing passions.

2. How:

- Develop a strategic plan: Determine how you will achieve your goals for creating a legacy and improving your health and happiness. Outline actionable strategies and practices.

- Creating a legacy: How will you build and leave your legacy?
    - Impact projects: Engage in initiatives or projects that align with your values and contribute positively to others. This could include mentoring, philanthropy or community service.
    - Documenting your story: Share your experiences, insights and lessons through writing, speaking or other forms of communication.
    - Building relationships: Foster strong connections with family, friends and colleagues to ensure your influence extends through your relationships.
    - Health and happiness: How will you enhance your wellbeing?
    - Health practices: Implement a balanced diet, regular exercise, sufficient sleep and stress management techniques.
    - Happiness practices: Incorporate activities and habits that bring joy and fulfilment, such as hobbies, social interactions and mindfulness.
    - Personal growth: Engage in continuous learning and personal development to enrich your life and maintain motivation.

3. When:

- Set a schedule for implementation: Specify when you will implement your strategies and track your progress. Consistency and timing are essential for achieving your goals.
- Implementation schedule: When will you work on your legacy and wellbeing?
    - Daily: Integrate small, consistent actions into your daily routine, such as healthy eating, exercise and engaging in positive interactions.
    - Weekly: Set aside time weekly to focus on legacy-building activities, such as working on projects or connecting with others. Review your health and happiness practices to ensure they align with your goals.
    - Monthly: Evaluate your progress toward your legacy and wellbeing goals. Adjust your strategies as needed and set new milestones for the coming month.

By focusing on the what, how and when of creating a lasting legacy and enhancing your health and happiness, you craft a clear, actionable roadmap to achieve your most meaningful aspirations. This formula empowers you to make intentional, purposeful decisions daily, ensuring your efforts align with your values and goals. When you commit to this holistic approach, you're not just improving your physical health—you're building a life rich with purpose, fulfilment and lasting happiness.

Remember to stay grounded in the fundamentals to build the life you want. These are the pillars that will support your success in the long term:

- **Exercise:** It is non-negotiable. Your exercise plan should target all four zones of fitness. Stay committed to tracking your progress, understanding your numbers and being consistent throughout the year. Aim for at least 45 out of 52 weeks of dedication to this element of your wellbeing.

- **Nutrition:** Your body thrives on variety. Consume a wide range of nutrient-dense foods (think colours and diversity), meet your macronutrient goals and ensure sufficient protein intake (2 g/kg of body weight). Portion control and hydration are crucial—aim for 150 mL of water every waking hour to keep your body functioning at its best.

- **Personalised blueprint:** Consistent and regular reviews are key to long-term success. Your blueprint should be tailored to your needs and constantly evolve based on progress and feedback. Track your measurements and progress—if you measure it, you can manage it. And do not forget to incorporate the things that bring you joy, whether hobbies, relationships or simply taking time for what makes you feel alive.

Now, it's time to act and build your desired life. Embrace this framework and make it a lifelong commitment. With dedication, consistency and a clear plan, you can create a future full of optimal health, happiness and the kind of legacy you want to leave behind. Here is to a life of wellbeing, satisfaction and enduring fulfilment. Let the journey begin!

Remember, life is a game; you make the rules.

Much Love,

TORY
#THEHEALTHBLOKE

www.torytrewhitt.com.au

info@torytrewhitt.com.au

REFERENCES

Basso, J.C. & Suzuki, W.A. (2017). 'The effects of acute exercise on mood, cognition, neurophysiology and neurochemical pathways: A review,' *Brain Plasticity* (Amsterdam, Netherlands), vol. 2, no. 2, pp. 127–152.

Bruce, A., Johnson, A., Lewis, J., Morgan, D. & Raff, M. (2014). *Molecular Biology of the Cell*, Taylor & Francis Group, Oxford.

Calvani, R., Joseph, A.M., Adhihetty, P.J., Miccheli, A., Bossola, M., Leeuwenburgh, C., Bernabei, R. & Marzetti, E. (2013). 'Mitochondrial pathways in sarcopenia of ageing and disuse muscle atrophy,' *Biological Chemistry*, vol. 394, no. 3, pp. 393–414.

Hanaway, P. (2024). How do stress and inflammation contribute to chronic disease? IFM, The Institute for Functional Medicine. Available at: https://www.ifm.org/news-insights/stress-inflammation-and-the-functional-medicine-model/ (Accessed: 14 November 2024).

Holt-Lunstad, J., Smith, T.B., Baker, M., Harris, T. & Stephenson, D. (2015). 'Loneliness and social isolation as risk factors for mortality: A meta-analytic review,' *Perspectives on Psychological Science*, vol. 10, no. 2, pp. 227–237.

'How much protein do you need every day?' (2015). Harvard Health. Available at: https://www.health.harvard.edu/blog/how-much-protein-do-you-need-every-day-201506188096

Kornrich, S., Brines, J. & Leupp, K. (2013). 'Egalitarianism, housework and sexual frequency in marriage,' *American Sociological Review*, vol. 78, no. 1, pp. 26–50. doi:10.1177/0003122412472340.

Langa, K.M. (2018). 'Cognitive ageing, dementia and the future of an ageing population,' in *Future Directions for the Demography of Ageing: Proceedings of a Workshop*, National Academies Press (US).

Lorenz, T. & Van Anders, S. (2014). 'Interactions of sexual activity, gender and depression with immunity,' *The Journal of Sex Medicine*, vol. 11, no. 4, pp. 966–979.

Malik, S., Xavier, S., Soch, A., Younesi, S., Yip, J., Slayo, M., Barrientos, R.M., Sominsky, L. & Spencer, S.J. (2024). 'High-fat diet and ageing-associated memory impairments persist in the absence of microglia in female rats,' *Neurobiology of Ageing*, vol. 140, pp. 22–32.

Martone, A., Marzetti, E., Calvani, R., Picca, A., Tosato, M., Santoro, L., Giorgio, A., Nesci, A., Sisto, A., Santoliquido, A. & Landi, F. (2017). 'Exercise and protein intake: A synergistic approach against sarcopenia,' *BioMed Research International*. Available at: https://www.researchgate.net/publication/313251568_Exercise_and_Protein_Intake_A_Synergistic_Approach_against_Sarcopenia

'Overweight and obesity' (n.d.). Australian Institute of Health and Welfare. Available at: https://www.aihw.gov.au/reports/overweight-obesity/overweight-and-obesity/contents/overweight-and-obesity (Accessed: 12 November 2024).

Thalacker-Mercer, A.E., Fleet, J.C., Craig, B.A., Carnell, N.S. & Campbell, W.W. (2007). 'Inadequate protein intake affects skeletal muscle transcript profiles in older humans,' *The American Journal of Clinical Nutrition*, vol. 85, no. 5, pp. 1344–1352.

Torres, S.J. & Nowson, C.A. (2007). 'Relationship between stress, eating behaviour and obesity,' *Nutrition*, vol. 23, no. 11–12, pp. 887–894.

www.ingramcontent.com/pod-product-compliance
Lightning Source LLC
Chambersburg PA
CBHW061725070526
44583CB00024B/3012